WALLABY

Yoga Moves

with Alan Finger

Alan Finger and Lynda Gellis Guber
Photographs by Norman Seeff

A Wallaby Book
Published by Simon & Schuster, Inc.
New York

Caution: Before starting this, or any other, exercise program, it is advisable to check with your physician.

Published by Wallaby Books
A Division of Simon & Schuster, Inc.
Simon & Schuster Building
1230 Avenue of the Americas
New York, New York 10020

Designed by Judy Allan

WALLABY and colophon are registered trademarks of Simon & Schuster, Inc.

First Wallaby Books printing May 1984
10 9 8 7 6 5 4 3 2 1

Manufactured in the United States of America
Printed and bound by Halliday Lithograph

Library of Congress Cataloging in Publication Data

Finger, Alan, date
Yoga moves with Alan Finger.

"A Wallaby book."
1. Yoga, Hatha.   I. Guber, Lynda Gellis.   II. Title.
RA781.7.F56   1984   613.7'046   83-20399
ISBN: 0-671-50064-3

Acknowledgments

To my husband, Peter Guber, who freely and generously gave of his time, patience, energy, love and total support. I love you. And to my daughters, Jodi and Elizabeth, who are always showing me the way and keeping me in line. I'm so happy I have you.

And of course, my love and gratitude to a very special person in my life, my teacher, Yogi Alan Finger. With him I have fully experienced that "the joy is in the process." And to his wife, Jaki, who has been a saint through all our hard work and collaboration.

To my parents Abe and Mussie Gellis, who started me on my journey.

Thanks to my friends Lynda Obst, Carole Isenberg, and Joclyn Zaretsky for their support and inspiration.

To Norman Seeff for his great pictures. To Lin Oliver, who stood by us all the way and made *Yoga Moves* possible.

To my brother Henry Gellis, whose light and love are always present, and who introduced me to Alan.

To David Winters for sharing my vision in the making of *Yoga Moves* and his endless support.

My very special thanks to my brother Sammy Gellis, who taught me that life was a gamble—so why not go for it. Although he is no longer with me his smile and glow will be felt forever.

And to everyone involved in the making of *Yoga Moves,* I thank you.

Lynda Gellis Guber

Dedication

This is for all the people who have contributed their time, energy, and love.

Thanks, Lynda, for putting so much time and energy into writing this book and for having the patience to bring out the essence of my teachings and techniques. Eternal love to you.

To Peter Guber, for clearing my way and making it all possible.

To my Father, Mani, for showing me the light.

To Jaki, my wife, for being there with strength and direction.

To Tevya and Deva, my children, for joy and inspiration.

To Rod Striker, for being so respectful and supportive.

To Norman Seeff, for the incredible photographs and endless support.

To Louise Levin and Keith Williamson, thank you for your help.

You are all part of a great experience and I thank you.

Alan Finger

Contents

I was born in Johannesburg, South Africa, in 1946, to a father who was shell-shocked in the war. Experiencing insufferable pain, both mental and physical, he turned to drugs and alcohol without relief. At the age of seven, I was a mess. I suffered palpitations, stomach flutters, lightheadedness. Since then, I've desperately searched for a cure through the scientific approaches, without any results. I was a compulsive eater at age fifteen, weighing in at 265 pounds.

By happenstance, my father encountered a yogi, Yogananda, who assisted him in transforming his life. Freed from pain and suffering, he dedicated himself to becoming a great master of Tantra Yoga.

Unhappy, frustrated, and fed up with life, at sixteen I decided to follow my father's footsteps and began the study of yoga and meditation. Within three months I lost 100 pounds and began to unfold the sensitive, artistic, centered person within me. This was a miracle. This profound change in my being made inevitable my choice to become a yoga master.

I studied with many Indian masters who toured through South Africa, and today have adapted my teachings to a Western life-style.

Settling in Los Angeles, California, I opened the Yoga Tantra Institute in West Hollywood, and began my teachings.

I do not seek a following. I teach people to become their own masters. I don't teach one to follow or to look for a master. I am a yogi-raj—a master of yoga, and I can teach people to become the master so that they may learn to help themselves.

Tantra Yoga involves physical and mental therapies, clearing one's mind far deeper than most other therapies or disciplines. It offers physical and mental growth, simultaneously. This form of yoga brings you to an understanding of yourself in an amazingly short period of time. Everyone wants to know how to find peace, strength, and clarity without the use of crutches. The practice of yoga offers just that.

Exposure in several national magazines and on television talk shows and the urging of my pupils, including numerous Hollywood celebrities, helped me decide to undertake this book of special techniques as a natural outgrowth of my commitment.

Yogi-raj Alan Finger

Yoga works—it really works.

Yoga, something I knew nothing about several years ago, has changed my life today. Alan Finger started teaching my husband Peter and me yoga for a specific reason. Peter had a painful lower-back problem that was incapacitating him. This energetic, vital man had been flat on his back for months.

Ready to try anything, having spent a lot of money on doctors for physical therapy—not to mention the time and energy involved—we began yoga. In one month, to my amazement and his, Peter was better than ever. This daily process of stretching, bending, balancing, and toning the body worked a miracle!

From then on yoga became part of my life and so did Alan. There was something in his attitude about life, the way he dealt with people, his ability to let go and move on. He was a yogi and a contemporary Western man. He brought a sense of humor to it all, a feeling of accomplishment and fun, inspiring me to want to succeed.

I began looking forward to my morning yoga sessions with Alan and on my own. Yoga became part of my daily routine, a quiet time for Peter and me to be together.

What began as a remedy for Peter became a way of life for me.

It was not long after I made my yoga commitment that people noticed changes in me. They asked if I was doing something different. My appearance changed. I seemed calmer, more focused and youthful-looking. I felt the differences in my body. I found yoga kept my body in shape without other forms of exercise. This amazed me!

With yoga I was working on my body and quieting my mind at the same time. Changes occurred in my relationships, my work and my day-to-day activities. I began to feel an inner peace, an inner glow.

I lead a very hectic life and that hasn't changed. What has changed is the way I deal with it. I am able to balance out the pieces and appreciate the fullness of it.

Wanting to share my discovery with others, I began teaching friends, peers, and children.

Having worked together to help me master yoga to a certain degree, Alan Finger and I decided to bring his unique teachings to a wider audience. We bring you *Yoga Moves,* a direct outgrowth of our desire to share this most ancient form of exercise with you.

We have put time, energy, thought, and lots of love into our work. We hope you enjoy *Yoga Moves.*

Lynda Gellis Guber

Introduction

In a world that is charged with tension and anxiety, we are all seeking a secret potion for good health and inner peace.

Yoga, the most ancient system of healing, toning, and rejuvenating your body, is this magic formula. It recognizes that a vital, healthy mind is the prerequisite for life's journey.

Alan Finger has immersed himself in the ancient forms of hatha and tantra yoga for twenty-two years, and has created a new kind of workout called "Yoga Moves."

Alan says, "Deep within each one of us is a strong, inspiring, healing force. A joy for life, waiting to be tapped."

It requires both inspiration and perspiration, and proves finally that *enlightenment isn't serious.*

The perspiration in Yoga Moves comes from the series of movements designed to stretch, strengthen, and align your body. The inspiration is achieved during the moments between poses where you allow your body and mind to adjust so that each posture flows continuously into the next, with the spaces in between being equally important.

Yoga Moves is not a contest. Just do the best you can. Each body has its own limitations. Work toward realizing your own perfections and recognizing your unique beauty.

Like any exercise, the more disciplined you are the more fulfilling the results. Yoga Moves deals with the whole human being. It is a process of aligning one's body, mind and spirit. You learn that the breath is your metronome. Yoga Moves requires the combination of proper breathing and physical movement in order to achieve success. What you first need to bring to Yoga Moves is your commitment. Anyone can do yoga. You are not too old, young, short, tall, skinny, or fat to experience the benefits of yoga. Modern life has become sedentary with processed foods and high anxiety. If you want to live to your fullest potential, you have to do something about it.

If you still want to jog, bicycle, play tennis, swim, or lift weights—great! Yoga Moves will only enhance your agility in these activities. There are no quick fixes, little white pills, or mechanical contraptions—just you and this wonderful machine called the human body, which only you can keep in shape. There's no trade-in.

If it's difficult at first, start slowly. A few moves done correctly will build the proper foundation.

Yoga Moves is presented in a complete one-hour format. As a beginner, or if your time is limited, the first half hour can be done as a complete unit. There is also a 15-minute routine and a quickie pick-up energizer.

Make the commitment and keep it. We all have time. There are no excuses.

Practice any time: In the morning, to energize and start the day; at night for a peaceful sleep, or even at lunch time to center yourself for the rest of the day. Nourish your entire body, not just your stomach.

Yoga's very best qualities are available to you.

Let's move into yoga.

Part One

How the Yogi Sees It

Yoga, Beauty and Youth

Yoga treats beauty from the inside out. Physical well-being is the world's perfect cosmetic.

Women and men spend millions of dollars annually on creams and lotions that promise glowing, radiant complexions. They could save a lot of time, disappointment and money if they realized that what goes on top of the skin is not as important as what goes on beneath it. The most effective cosmetic for a glowing, healthy complexion is good circulation and detoxification of the body. Yoga Moves, in conjunction with proper breathing, creates increased circulation, enriches the skin tissues, and purifies the blood.

Yoga Moves stretches out your body by working on the spine, the central core of the nervous system. A supple spine is essential for maintaining a youthful appearance.

Gravity is constantly pulling down on our body. By standing upside down (as in the inverted poses), we let the body get a reversal of gravitational pull.

Yoga Moves create space in between the vertebrae, realigning your spine. Pay close attention during the poses not to slouch or collapse at the spine. It will keep that life force called *prana* flowing through your body and rejuvenating it.

You have only one body to get you through this entire lifetime. So take care of it. Nurture it. Feed it. Exercise it and listen to it.

A flexible body is a youthful body. Men, in general, are less flexible than women. Athletic men often put too much emphasis on developing certain parts of the body, allowing other areas to become stiff with age. As we do the postures we stretch our bodies, increase our flexibility, and strengthen our muscles.

In yoga, we stand, move, and sit with awareness, until it becomes a natural part of us. Good posture goes hand in hand with beauty and youthfulness.

The Difference Between Yoga and Exercise

In Yoga Moves we love ourselves into shape, not beat ourselves into shape.

Yoga Moves is a series of poses specially designed to balance the energy of your entire body, mind, and nervous system.

Each move is an exercise in itself with the specific purpose of repairing and maintaining individual parts of your body. However, taking one pose to benefit one alignment is limiting. The purpose of yoga is to benefit the whole body, not just its parts.

Properly done the physical workout is equal to any exercise program.

However, Yoga Moves is *a personal workout of the body and the mind.*

As you hold the pose your entire body is strengthened and toned. At the same time you become aware of your restless thoughts and recognize feelings locked inside you. The longer the pose is held the more you build your strength and your mind quiets down.

As you begin to break through your barriers you set up new goals, so that each workout is a new experience in growth.

Breathing

Let your breath be your guide.

Air is our most important food. Because breathing is involuntary, we tend to ignore it, forgetting that the breath and mind work together.

Whatever state of mind you're in, your breath will follow. When doing postures let your breath be your guide. If it becomes harsh and jerky, you're overdoing it. Always keep your breath full and even. When you first begin you may breathe in through your nose and out through your mouth. However, with practice, learn to inhale and exhale only through your nose.

Strong lungs and good full breathing are a sign of abundant energy.

When doing a posture, there is a tendency to hold your breath. Be aware of this and keep your breath moving. While holding the posture, breathe evenly, smoothly and deeply.

Breathing is the key to understanding *prana*—our life force.

Relaxation

A lost art in a society going 100 mph. Stop!

Relaxation is the sum total of quieting your body and your mind. It is the ability to transcend thought, time, and space, reaching a moment of inner peace, a moment between two thoughts.

Most people consider relaxation to be an occupation such as reading a book, watching TV, going to a movie, the beach, walking a dog. Although these activities are therapeutic, true relaxation only takes place when there is a total stillness in one's body and mind. When the brain rhythm is quieted, the healing and recharging process begins. As soon as mental activity begins, relaxation ends. It is for this reason that the yogi calls the relaxation process the Corpse Pose.

Meditation—An Inner Journey

Meditation takes you on a journey to a world of unlimited knowledge, joy, and healing, beyond the emotional and the intellectual. It brings you to a place of intuitive knowledge called wisdom.

The nature of the mind is restless. It constantly searches outside for happiness and fulfillment. Meditation is the art of getting the mind to be still and to explore the peace, joy, and inner wisdom that lie within every given moment.

When you sit to meditate you will begin to uncover a whole spectrum of feelings that are stored in your unconscious. Be patient and allow yourself time to release them.

Meditation and Healing

Think of your mind as a lake. If it is still, you can see clearly to the bottom. If it is choppy, you can't see what there is in its depth.

Meditation can produce a state of profound clarity. Whenever any form of energy is concentrated and focused, its power increases. For example, a laser beam is nothing more than focused light—the same energy we get from a household light bulb.

The same happens in meditation. You focus the power of your mind into one point so that all your energies are concentrated. When the mind becomes still you become aware of the blocks in your physical and mental body. Once you know where the blocks are, you can focus your attention on them and actually direct energy to them, releasing and opening them.

Research has been done on the physiological effects of the profound relaxation produced by meditation. Doctors have found that meditation done on a regular basis is beneficial to people with coronary heart disease, reducing high blood pressure and decreasing irregular heartbeat and muscular tension. They also have found fewer symptoms associated with anxiety, including headaches, nausea, rashes, diarrhea, mouth sores, insomnia, worrying, and nervous habits such as chewing pencils and biting fingernails.

One of the most important benefits of regular meditation is that it allows you to better maintain your equilibrium under stressful situations. It is not just that you are able to cope with stress better—situations simply do not bother you as much. Your well-being and equilibrium become less easily disturbed, not just while meditating but most of the time.

Meditation helps shift our attention from looking only at the goal—the future—to enjoying the process of what we are doing now—the present. Events are usually less stressful and more pleasurable when we focus on the process rather than on just the goal.

What is the process? It is simply being aware of and enjoying each moment. "Life is a process," says Dean Ornish, M.D., author of *Stress, Diet and Your Heart,* "not just a series of goals to be achieved."

Pain Versus Heightened Awareness

When practicing yoga, you may experience pain.

There are different kinds of pain. One pain is sharp and jarring, like a toothache. The pain that the yogis call "heightened awareness" is a release of tension in your muscles. This sensation disappears as you hold the pose; then as you adjust you can move deeper into the pose.

If you are experiencing pain in any posture, stop! Make sure you move into the posture slowly and correctly. If you are a beginner, don't expect too much too soon. The photographs are to be considered goals—models of what you might achieve after long practice. Never go beyond what your body tells you. You are using your total body in a way you never have before —there will be a natural resistance.

Diet

Most of us have learned to feed emotional needs with food. And so a large percentage of our eating is feeding our neuroses. We need to sort out our emotional problems away from the dining-room table. Postures, meditations, and visualizations are the techniques we offer you.

As you practice yoga more and more, you will begin to get a sense of the kinds of foods that your body needs to keep it in balance. It is because we are so unfamiliar with our own bodies that we go to others to find out what we need to stay fit.

Good nutrition is the foundation on which all good health is built.

The basic guidelines to a balanced diet:

> Low salt
> Low fat
> No processed sugars
> No red meats
> Fresh vegetables & fruits
> Caffeine—cut out or cut down
> Alcohol—cut out or cut down
> Water—eight glasses daily (detoxifies and cleanses
>   the body)
> No drugs
> No smoking

Read labels for ingredients and use your common sense.

It's okay to have a treat now and then. Remember, balance and moderation are the keys to good nutrition and a healthy state of being.

Dress

Most of us have learned to avoid what we don't want to see. So we have successfully learned to dress to hide our bodies.

Our pores absorb energy and excrete toxins. When doing yoga this process is tremendously accelerated. Therefore, it is best to wear light and comfortable clothing. Nonsynthetics are best, for they allow your skin to breathe.

The less you wear the more you see.

Environment

We perceive the world through our senses. Our environment stimulates different moods, emotions, and states of being. To enhance the effect of yoga, it's best to have a quiet place where you will not be disturbed. The room should be ventilated and on the warm side. A useful tool is a full-length mirror. A hard floor is best for standing postures and a carpet is best for floor postures.

Create your own world! Peace, joy and strength lie within you—make them part of your environment no matter where you are.

FingerPrints—How to Approach the Postures

1. Don't sacrifice form for range. Go only as far as you can.
2. Move in and out of poses slowly.
3. A posture is always built from the ground up. The ground or floor is your foundation.
4. Always begin by taking a full breath in and move into the posture on the exhalation.
5. Enjoy the moment between two breaths—it is the moment between two thoughts.
6. By relaxing and breathing fully while performing a posture, you will eliminate fatigue and feel re-energized.
7. Yoga Moves is not a competition.
8. Surrender into the pose.
9. Think and feel each pose.
10. Every time you do a pose feel as though it is the very first time you are attempting it.
11. Concentrate—if you snooze you lose.
12. Be patient! Your body will release and change.
13. Be happy within yourself and you will be happy with everything else. The joy is in the process.

Timing the Postures

The best way to time the holding of a posture is not by a clock. This will only create a break in your concentration. Some postures will be timed by counting the number of breaths you take while holding the position, others by counting up to 15. This will absorb you into the posture and the process.

Yoga Moves—The Four Routines

The complete series of postures lends itself to four formats: the full set, which takes about one hour; the first half, which takes about 30 minutes; the 15-minute routine, outlined below; and the Quickie routine. Each format can be used individually to learn yoga as well as for relaxation and meditation.

FIFTEEN-MINUTE ROUTINE:
Tadasan
Arm rotation
Tadasan
Arm extension
Tadasan
Blown Palm
Triangle
Fan
Tadasan
Sun Worship, 2 times
Bellows Breath
Relaxation

In the 15-minute routine, Tadasan are used in between the other moves for realignment. However, only hold them for 3 breaths.

QUICKIE ROUTINE:
If you're tired during the day and want a quick energizer, do the following moves:
Tadasan
Arm Rotation
Arm Extension
Sun Worship, 2 times

This is a process, not a one-shot deal. Every journey begins with but one step.

Part Two

Postures, Relaxation, Meditation

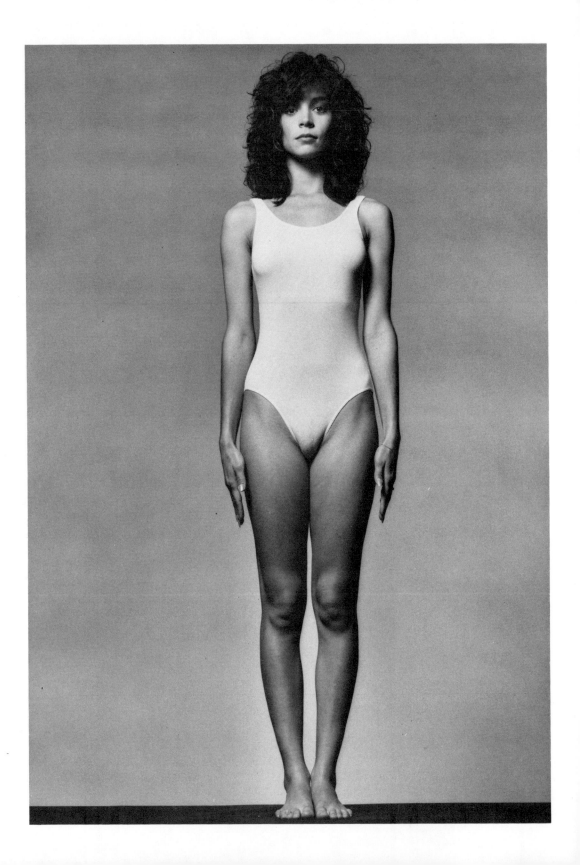

Tadasan

This is the basic yoga pose used in between each standing posture to realign and readjust your body.

Moves In:
 (1) Stand with feet together, big toes and heels touching and toes spread open. Distribute the weight evenly on the balls of both feet. Pull kneecaps up, tightening thighs; pinch seat tight together. Flatten abdominal wall, feel breastbone opening up and shoulders pulling back and relaxing down, as fingertips point downward, hands open.
 (2) Get the feeling of your spine lifting up, through the top back crown of your head, as if a string were pulling you up.
 (3) Keep face relaxed, eyes looking down at 45-degree angle. Breathe smoothly, holding the pose, eventually up to one minute.
 (4) Spread toes as much as possible, to create a broad foundation for balance.

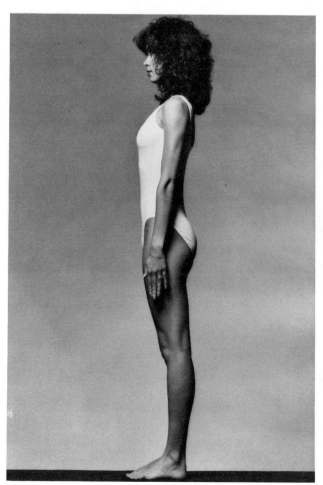
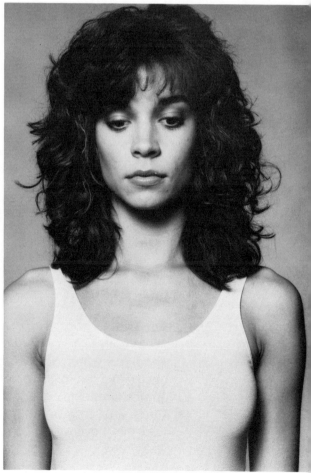

Moves Out:
> Never move out of the posture—only kidding. However, it does keep you walking tall, standing tall and thinking tall. So, remember to come back and practice Tadasan after each standing pose.

Be Aware: Do not arch your back; maintain smooth, even breathing.

Benefits: Teaches correct alignment of spine, which keeps you looking youthful. Excellent for tightening seat and thigh muscles. Remember to use it throughout your day to center yourself.

Arm Rotation

Moves In:
> (1) Stand with feet about two feet apart, turning them out to a 45-degree angle. Bend knees out to a half-squatting position so that they are in line with your ankles. Tighten thighs, pinch seat and keep spine tall.
>
> (2) Stretch arms out horizontally at shoulder level, palms of your hands down.
>
> (3) Circle your arms from the shoulder, 15 times forward and 15 times backward. Feel the movement begin from the shoulder joints. The rest of body remains stationary.

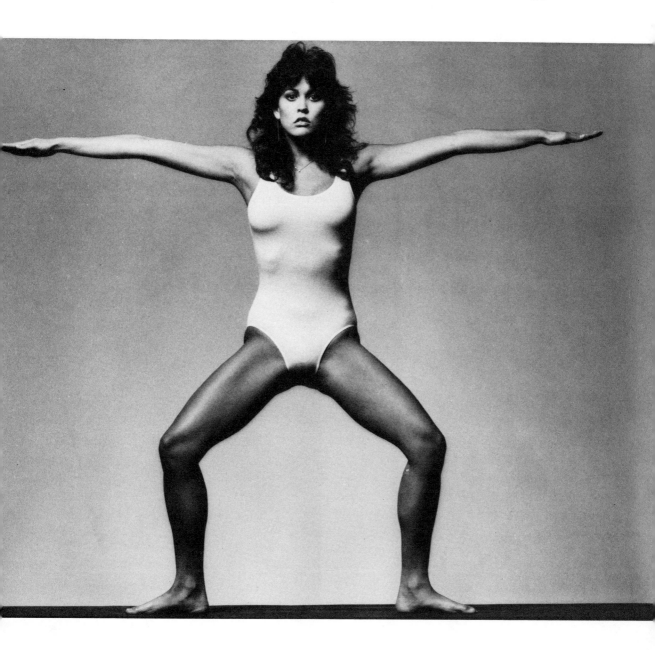

Moves Out:
     Bring arms down, straighten legs and step back into Tadasan.
Be Aware: Do not sway your spine back and forth. Keep your face relaxed—breathe evenly.
Benefits: Strengthens thighs, keeps seat firm, loosens deep tension from neck and shoulders, giving one a graceful appearance.

Arm Extension

Moves In:
(1) Stand facing a wall, an arm's-length away, your feet 15 inches apart.
(2) Place hands flat on the wall just above the level of your hairline, and extend seat back, feeling abdomen flat and spine stretched. Keep ears between biceps and feel chest expanding as shoulders open.
(3) Breathe smoothly and hold for 15 breaths.

Moves Out:
Tighten thighs and seat to stand up tall. Bring legs together into Tadasan and adjust.

Be Aware: Use stomach and thigh muscles. Don't sway your back. Breathe evenly through the posture.

Benefits: Keeps your spine straight, correcting curvature of the spine. Releases tension from chest, shoulders and arms. For women, it keeps the breasts firm.

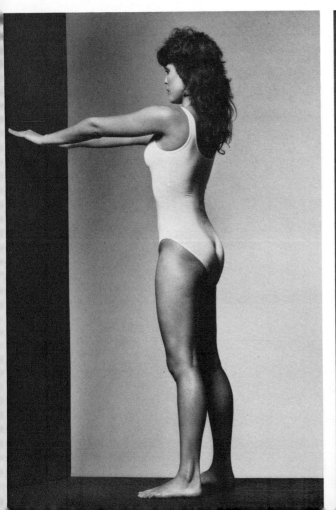
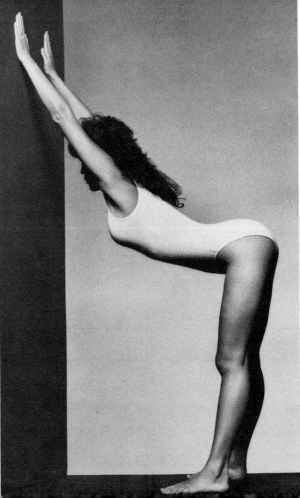

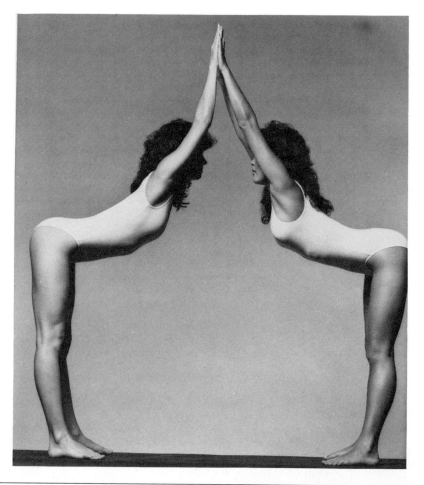

Arm Extension with Partner

Moves In:

(1) Stand facing partner with arms stretched out.

(2) Feet 15 inches apart.

(3) Place your palms on your partner's and press up, seat stretched and pushing out behind you.

(4) Keep your ears between your biceps with your neck flat, eyes looking down at a 45-degree angle. Hold the posture, building up to 15 to 20 breaths.

Moves Out:

(1) Tighten thighs and stand upright.

(2) Step back to Tadasan and take a full breath in through your nose and out through your mouth.

Be Aware: Use the strength of your abdomen and thighs to hold the posture. Let your hands balance you.

Benefits: The same as arm extension at the wall; however, this requires more strength to support yourself, as you cannot lean on your partner as you do on the wall.

Blown Palm

Moves In:
(1) Stand with feet together as in Tadasan. Raise your left arm into the air, palm facing the ceiling. Hold left wrist with right hand. Take a full breath in and stretch up. Stretch over to the right side from your waist; exhale. Keep torso facing forward. Don't twist! Breathe smoothly. Hold, building to 10 breaths.
(2) Repeat the posture on other side.

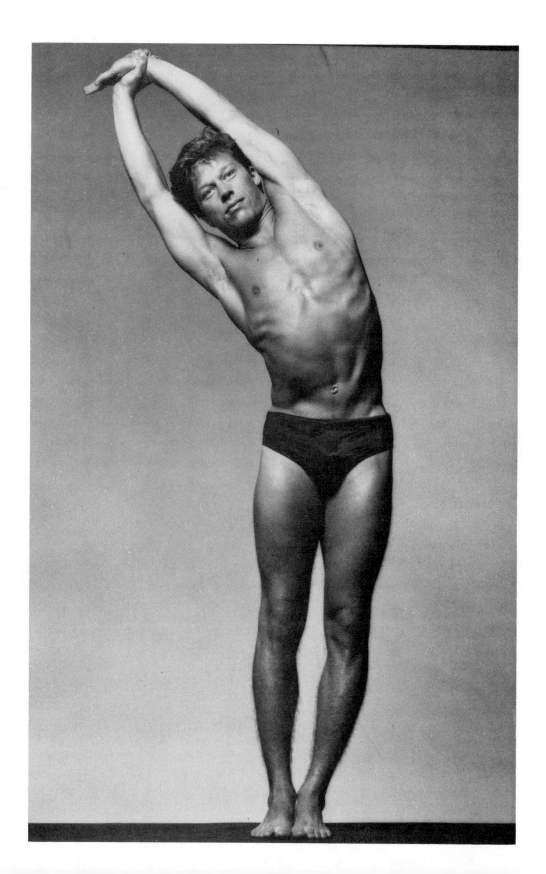

(3) Stretch arms above head with biceps beside ears and palms facing each other. Look between fingertips; tighten frontal thighs and seat. Take a full breath in stretching up as far as you can. On exhalation, bend back as far as is comfortable. Feel the bend in your shoulder blades, not in your lower back! Breathe through, building up to 10 breaths. Come back up tall; drop chin to chest.

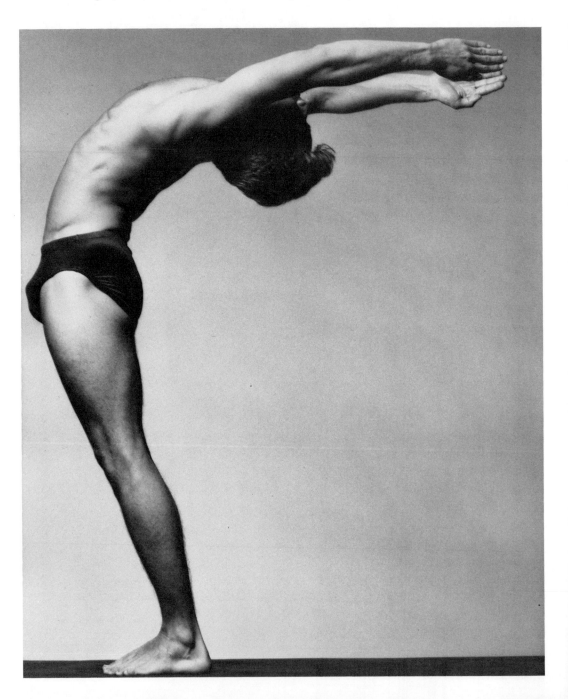

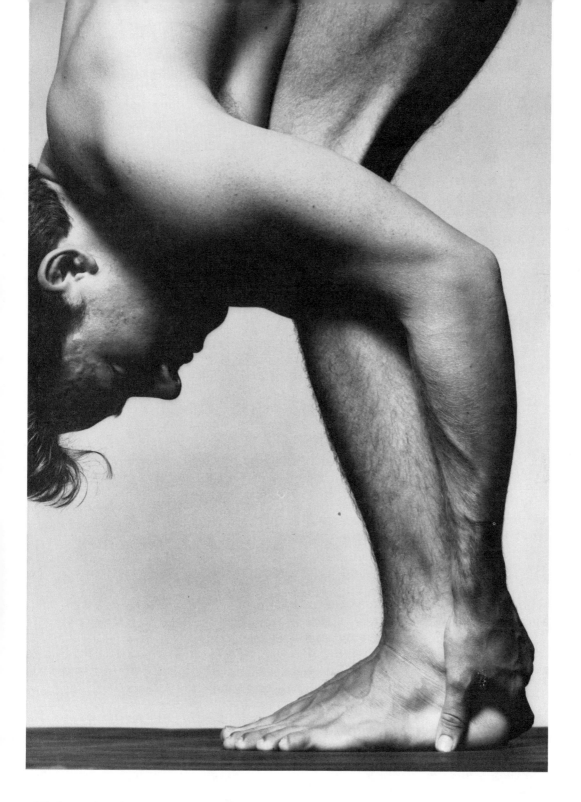

(4) Lowering hands down to sides, bend knees and grab ankles. Place thumbs on the floor beside your heels, elbows behind calves.

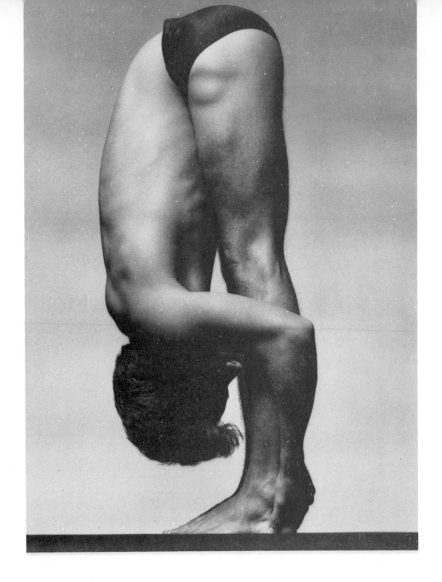

(5) Straighten your legs. Breathe through, building to 15 breaths.

Moves Out:

(1) Bend knees, using thighs and stomach to slowly stand tall, keeping seat muscles tight.

(2) Keep chin into neck and visualize one vertebra on top of the other as you come up. Allow your blood pressure to readjust. Breathe.

(3) Stand back into Tadasan.

Be Aware: In the backbend, do not bend into your lower back. Go as far as is comfortable, using thighs and seat muscles to project spine up and over. Breathe evenly. In the forward bend, keep your elbows behind your calves and work at pressing your seat up into the air as your legs straighten. From the forward bend, use your frontal thighs to pull yourself to an upright position.

Benefits: Stretches the spine, allowing blood to massage the spinal column, the center of the nervous system. Loosens and tones hips. Releases unconscious tension behind your legs.

Triangle

Moves In:

(1) Bring fingertips to touch in front of chest at shoulder height, with elbows bent out to the side. Bend your knees.

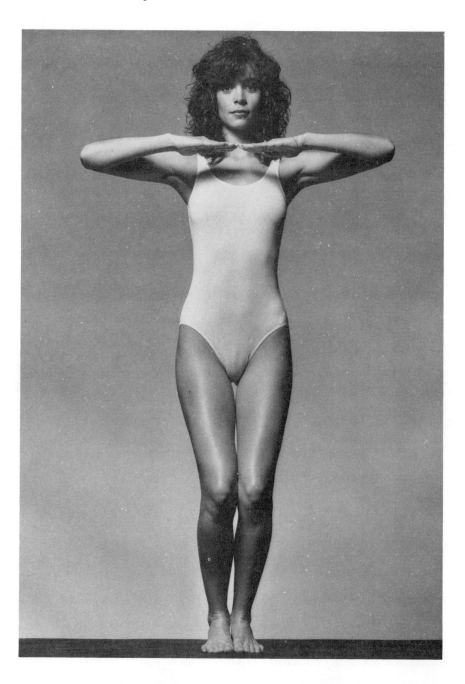

(2) Jump, feet 3 feet apart, arms out to the side.

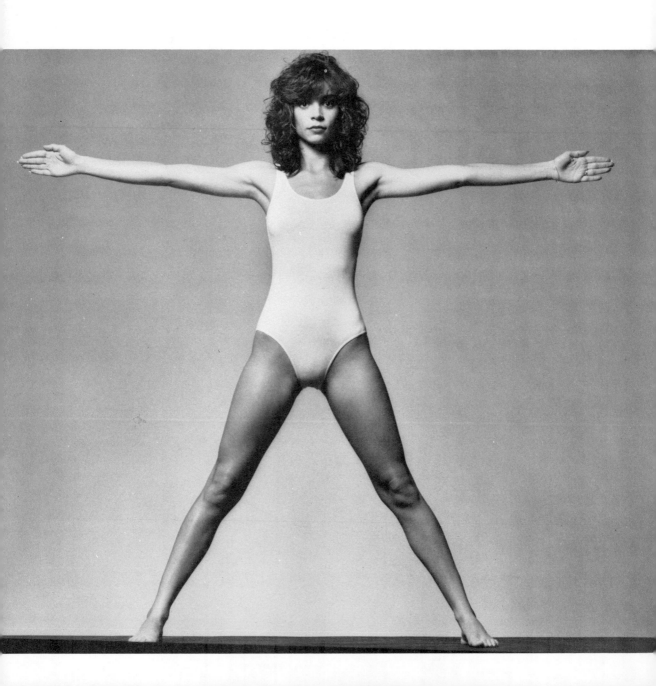

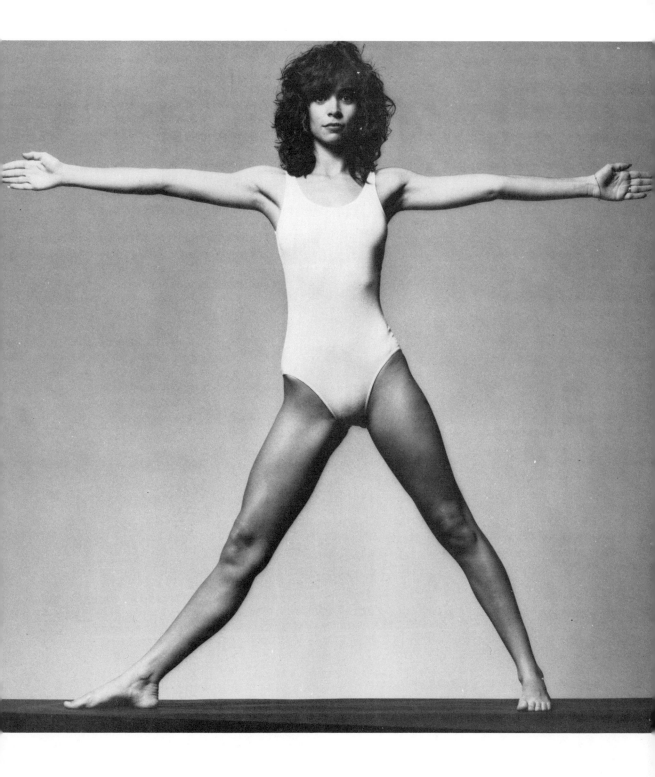

(3) Turn feet to the right, right foot 90 degrees from front, and left just slightly turned in. Breathe in, tightening thighs, and pull kneecaps up.

(4) As you exhale, stretch your torso out to the right side as far as possible, without turning hips.

(5) Move right hand down right leg as far as possible, to eventually have fingertips touching the floor. Look down to the foot on the floor and align your spine over right leg.

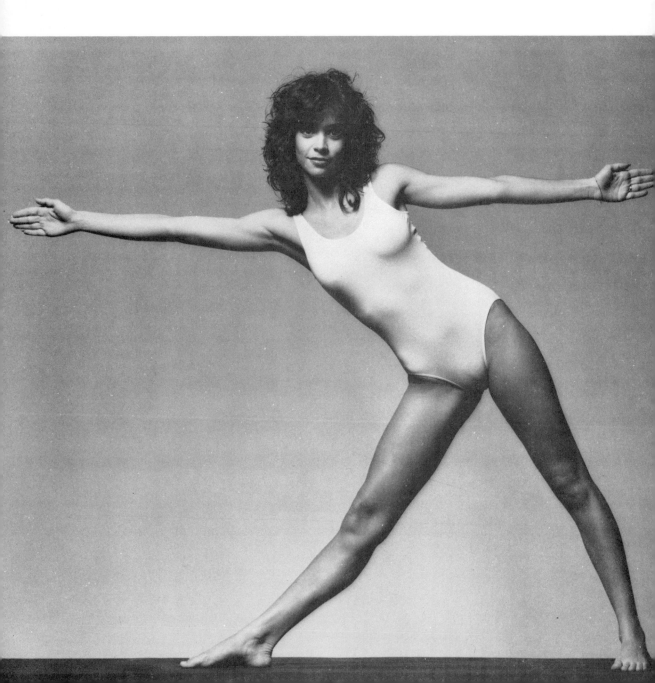

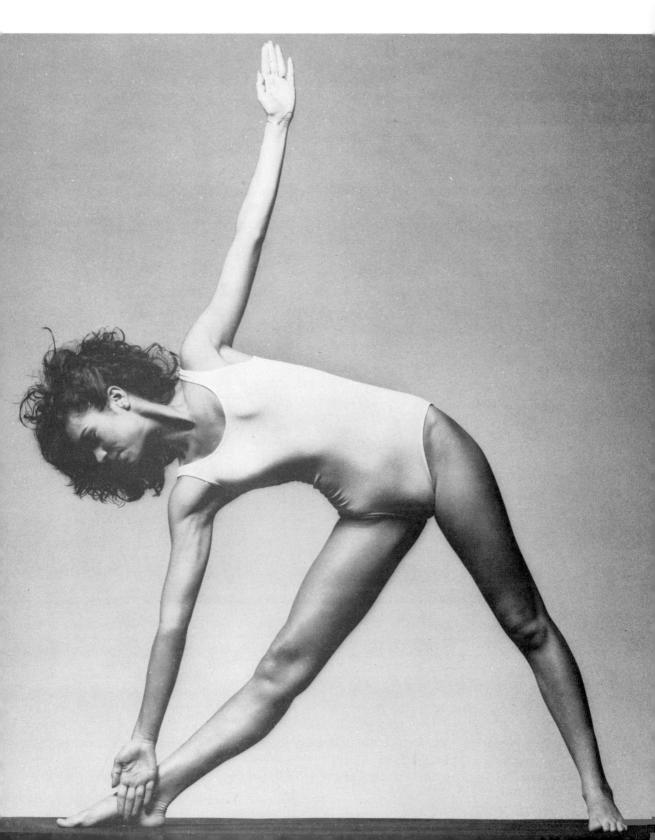

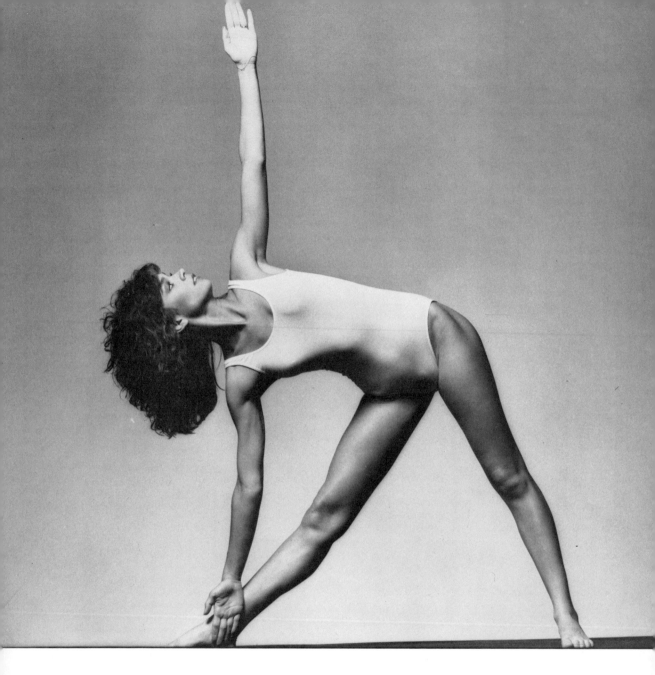

(6) Then slowly look up to your thumb in the air. Hold the posture, building up to 15 breaths.

Moves Out:

Tighten thighs, taking a breath in; on the exhalation come up. Keeping feet apart and facing forward, change angle of the feet to repeat on the other side. On completion, stand back into Tadasan.

Be Aware: Use your legs as the foundation of this posture, keeping your abdomen flat without twisting your body.

Benefits: Stretches your spine and strengthens your legs. Opens your hips and neck.

Triangle with Partner

Moves In:

(1) Stand back to back with partner, 6 inches apart, feet 3 feet apart. Both partners turn feet to the same side, one foot to a 90-degree angle from the front, and the other slightly turned in. Open arms out to the side and then intertwine yours with your partner's.

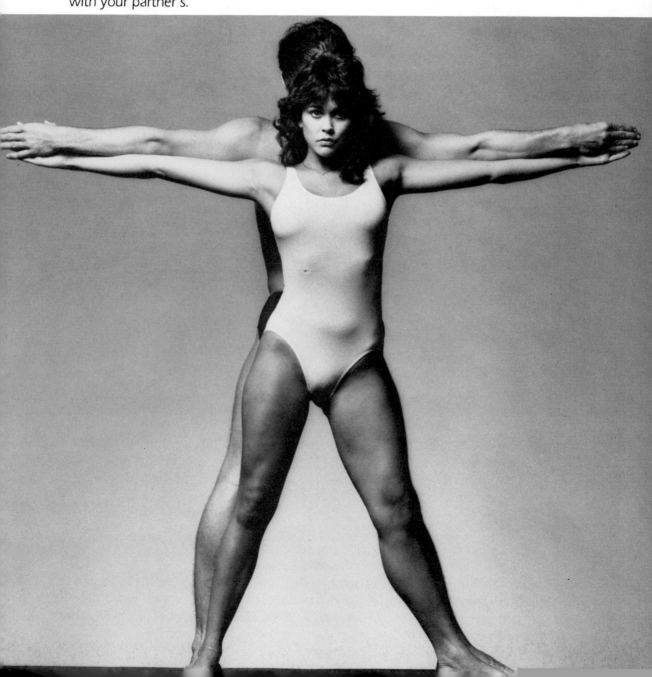

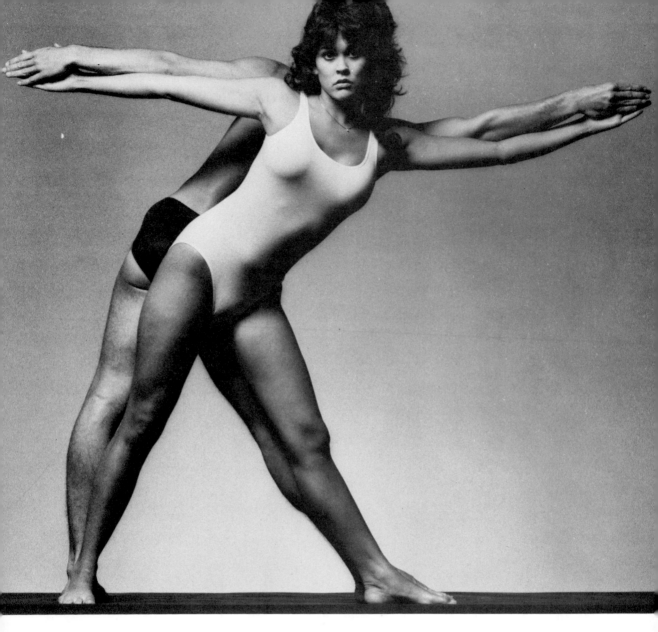

(2) Breathe in, tightening thighs, and pull kneecaps up. Breathe out. Stretch your-
    selves over to the side where the foot is turned to a 90-degree angle.
(3) Aim hands toward the floor, looking down at your foot. Slowly turn and look up
    at your hand in the air. Hold up to 30 seconds.
(4) Slowly come up, take a full breath in and exhale. Repeat on other side.

Moves Out:
(1) Slowly come up to a standing position; take a full breath.
(2) Release arms, feet together and into Tadasan.

Be Aware: Use your partner to align yourself. Feel your backs flat together.

Benefits: Tones all the muscles, especially those in your legs. To do this properly, you
must become attentive to all parts of your body simultaneously. You also become
sensitive to your partner's needs.

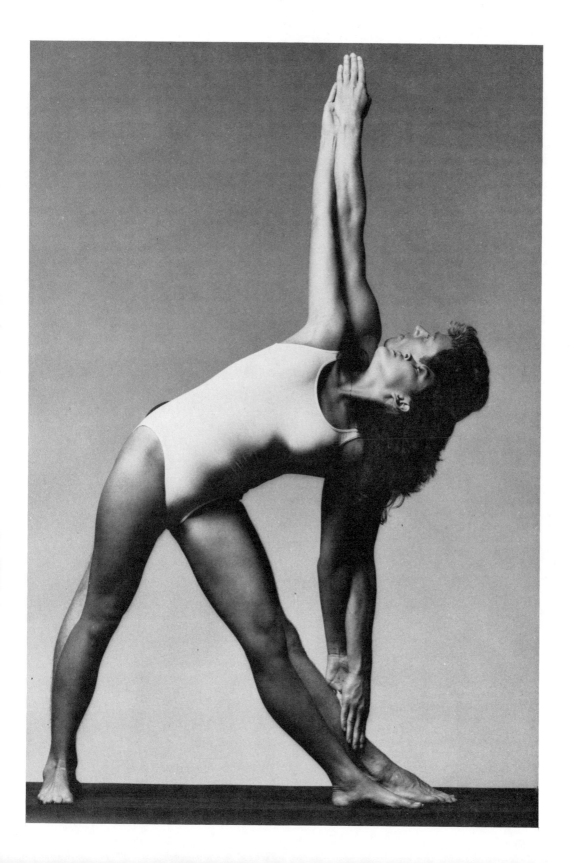

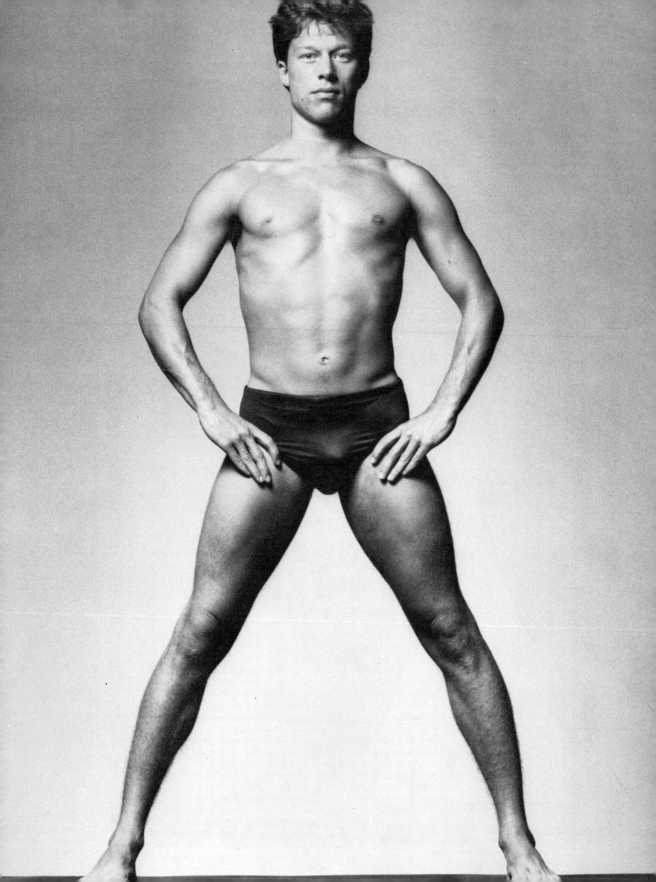

Fan

Moves In:

(1) Place hands along groin line, taking a full breath into the abdomen and expanding the breath into chest.

(2) Gently drop your head back.

(3) On the exhalation bend forward from hips.

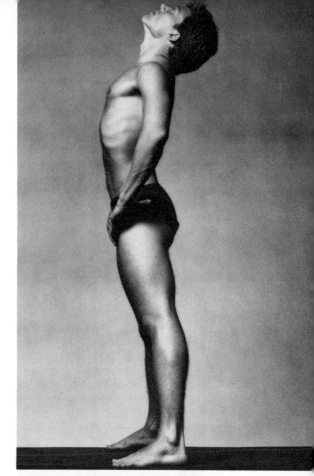

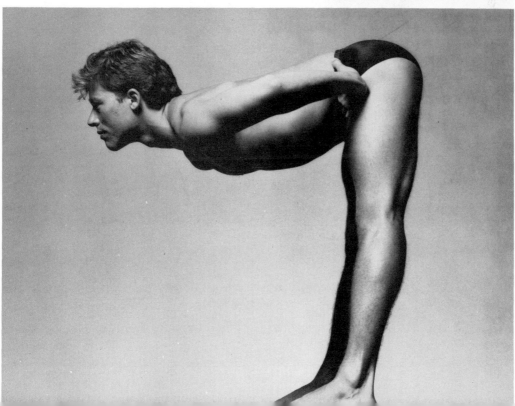

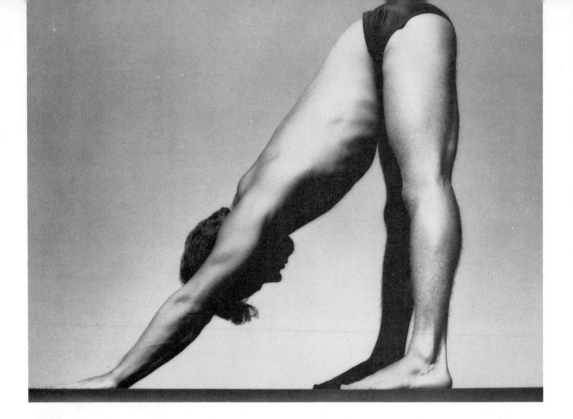

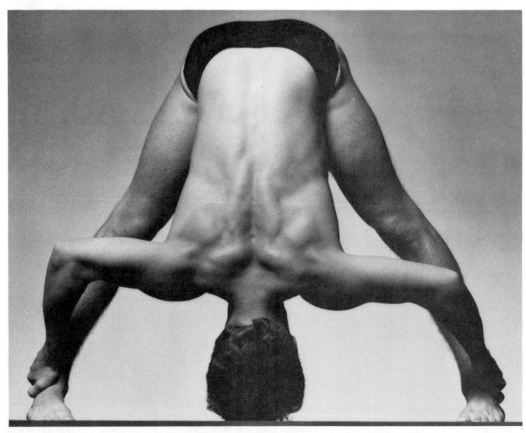

(4) Place hands on the floor and walk them out as far as possible, feeling the stretch from the seat to the fingertips.

(5) Release the stretch and grasp ankles with hands. Bend elbows out to the side, pulling hairline toward the floor between feet. Hold the pose, building up to 15 breaths.

Moves Out:

Walk hands up legs with a straight spine (thighs and seat tight). Keep chin tucked into neck and back parallel to floor. Clasp hands together behind neck, elbows straight out, and pull yourself to an upright position. When blood pressure adjusts bring head back to normal. Take a full breath, bring legs together into Tadasan.

Be Aware: Go only as far down as a straight spine permits. The stretch is in the back of your legs.

Benefits: Tightens thighs and seat muscles, lengthens spine, giving a youthful appearance. Releases tension from hamstrings behind legs, freeing hip structure. Releases unconscious tension from behind the legs.

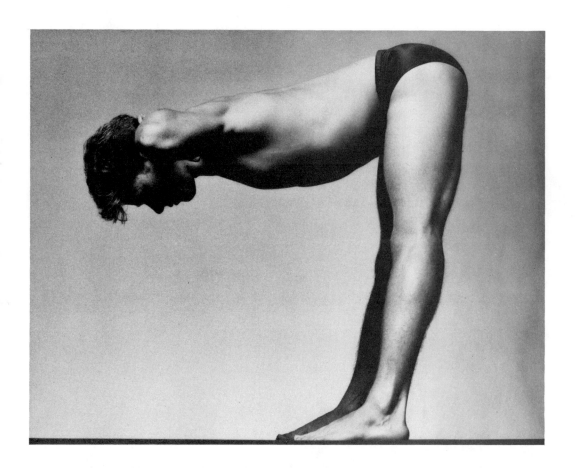

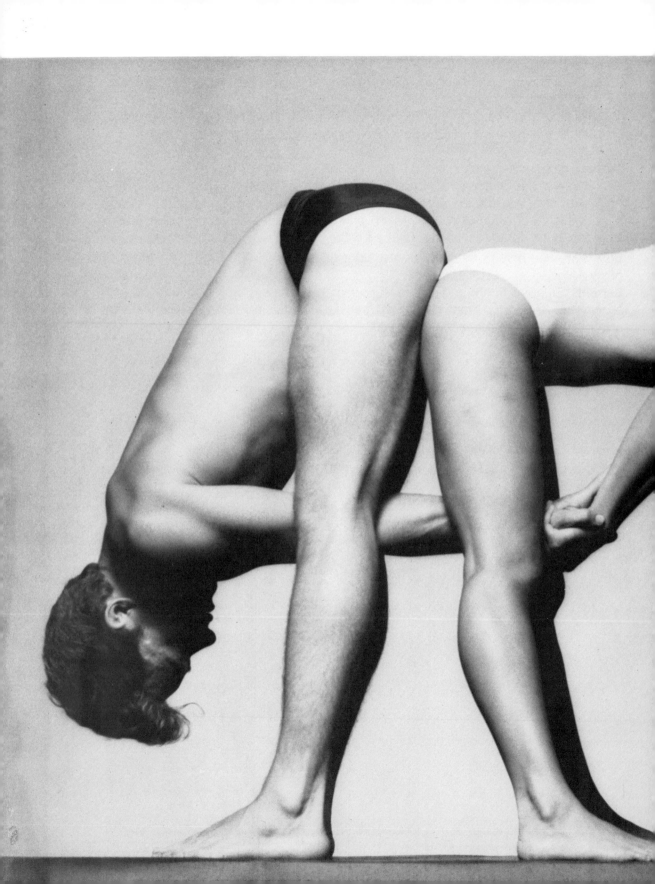

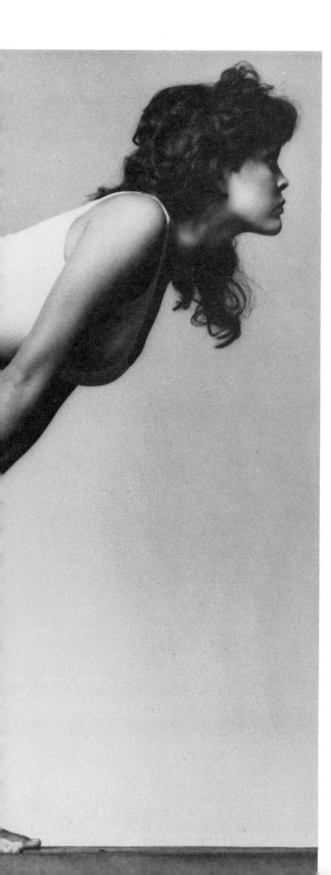

Fan with Partner

Moves In:

Stand back to back, 12 inches away from your partner, your feet 3 feet apart. Bend forward and stretch your hands between your legs to clasp each other's wrists. As one partner moves up, the other is pulled down. Move back and forth 3 times, taking enough time for each to get the stretch.

Moves Out:

Release each other's wrists and slowly come to stand up, with your chin into your chest. As your blood pressure adjusts, bring your head back to normal and stand into Tadasan.

Be Aware: Don't bend your spine. Keep your back straight.

Benefits: These are the same as in the fan pose; however, doing these moves with a partner intensifies the stretch.

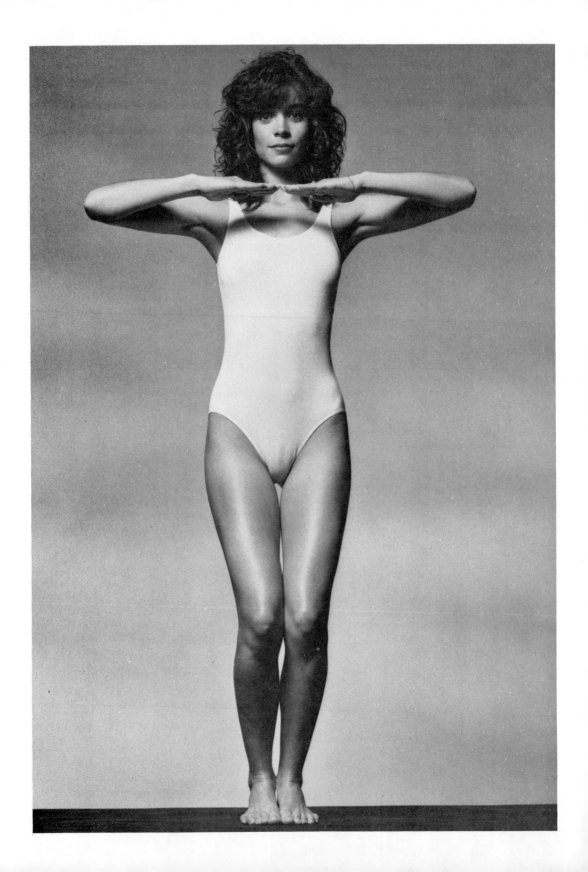

Worship Pose

Moves In:

(1) Standing in Tadasan, bring fingertips together in front of chest at shoulder level, elbows out to the side. Bend your knees.

(2) Jump, feet 3 feet apart, and open arms to the side.

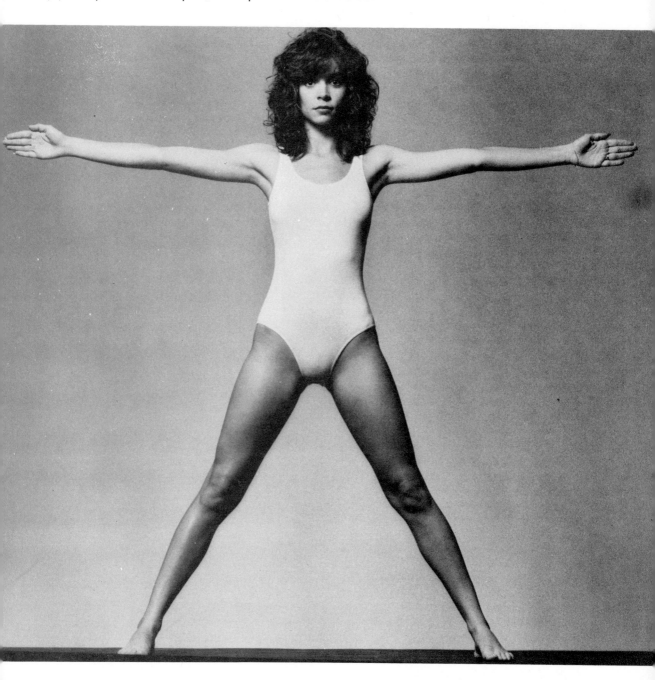

(3) Turn your feet to the right, right foot to a 90-degree angle from front and left foot just slightly turned in. Bend right leg to a right-angle position, keeping arms straight out to side (shoulder level).

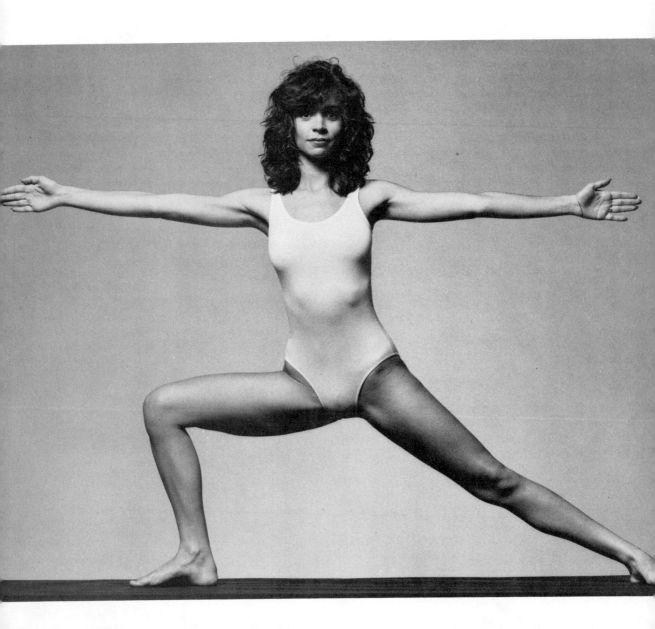

(4) Turn torso and head to look to right thumb.

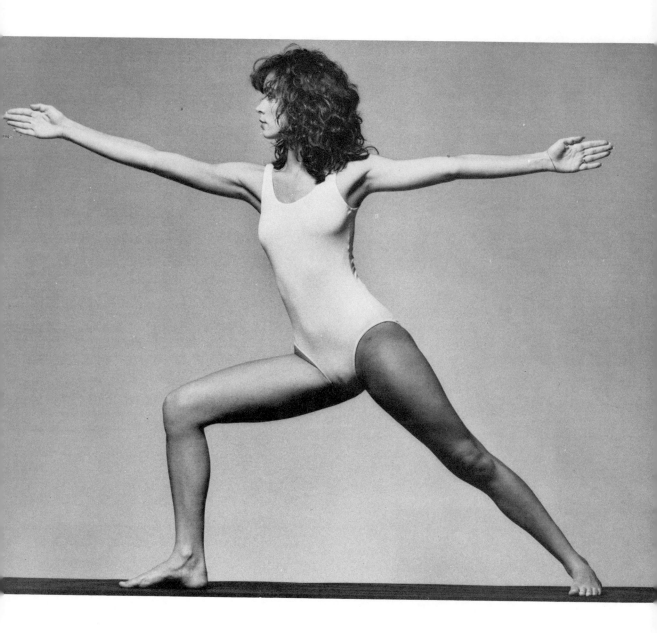

(5) Bring left arm parallel to right so that palms are facing each other.

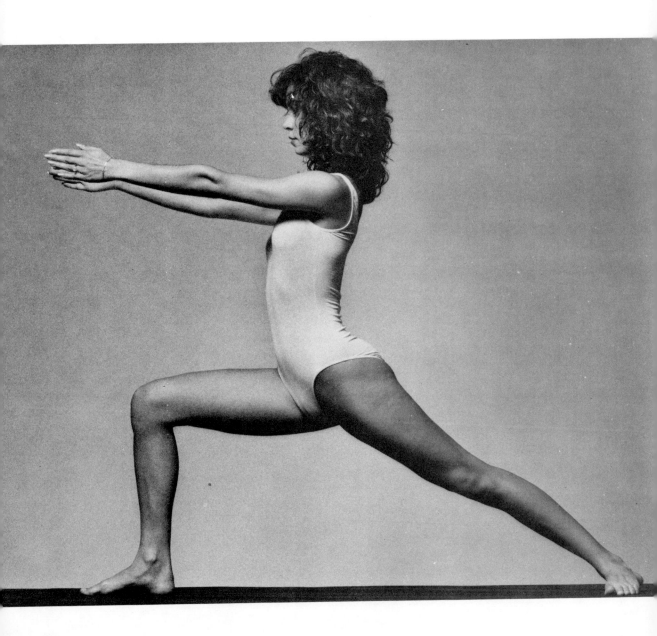

(6) Bring both hands up high above the head and look up between fingertips, stretching the torso long.

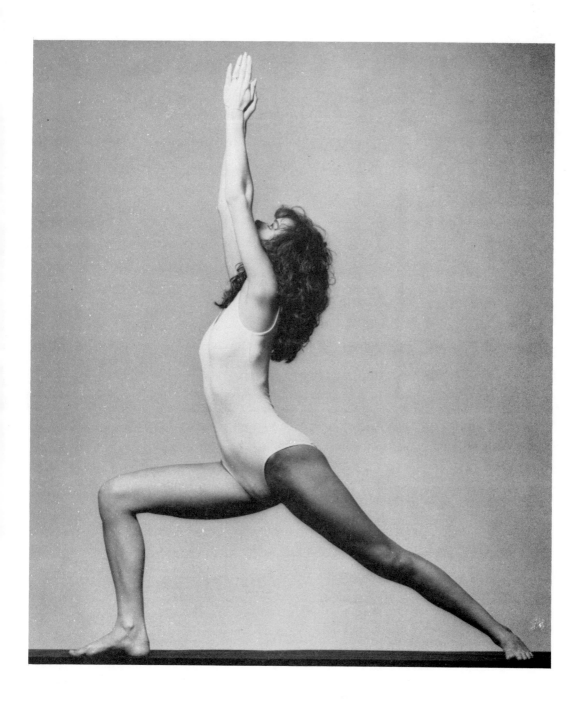

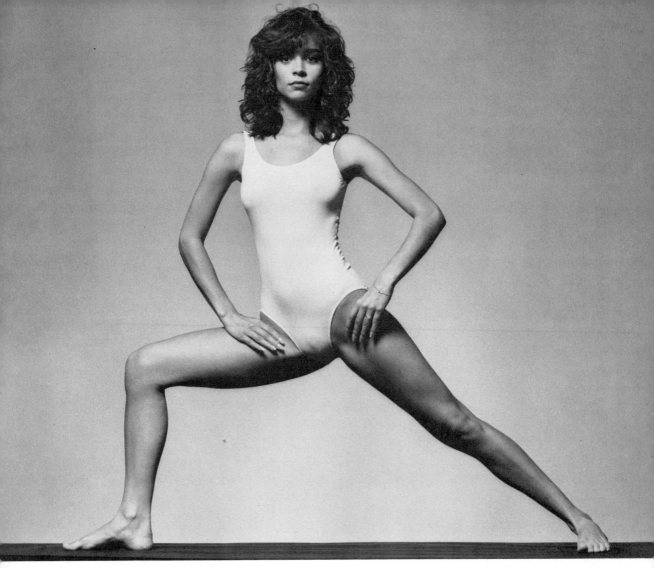

(7) Lower your arms and face front, taking 2 breaths. Turn feet to the left and repeat the posture.

Moves Out:
Stand back into Tadasan.

Be Aware: Use thighs, stomach and seat to project torso and spine into the stretch. Breathe evenly.

Benefits: Firms your thighs, creates concentration and determination.

Dancer

Moves In:
(1) Standing in Tadasan, rotate right arm outward so that inner elbow and palm face away from body. Bring up right foot and grab the inside of ankle with right hand. Raise left arm up into the air beside your head, palm facing forward.

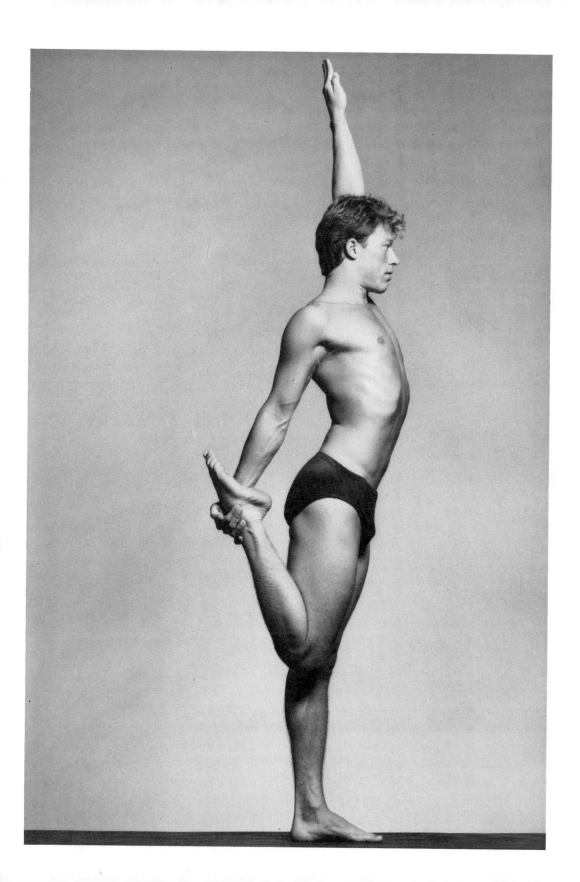

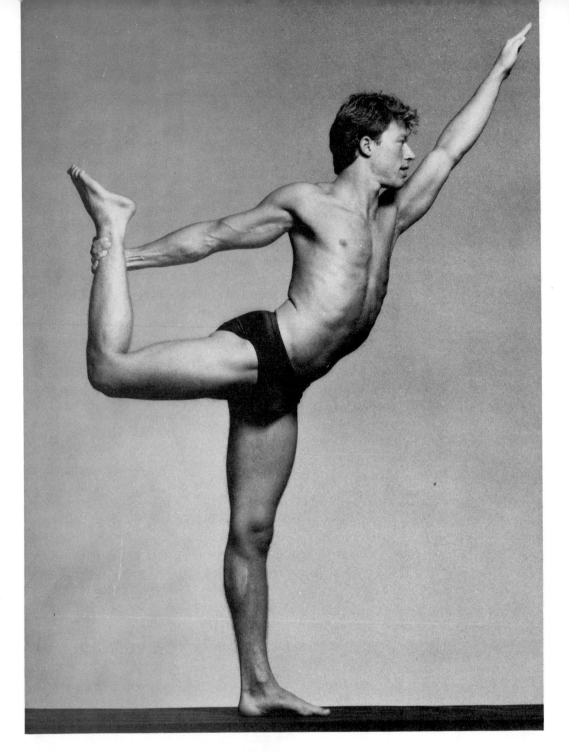

(2) Bend forward, keeping chest open, lowering the left arm forward and simultaneously raising your right leg behind you.

(3) Straighten your right leg as much as possible. Hold the posture, building up to 10 breaths.

Moves Out:

Lower the right leg, raising the left arm up into the air. Release foot back to the

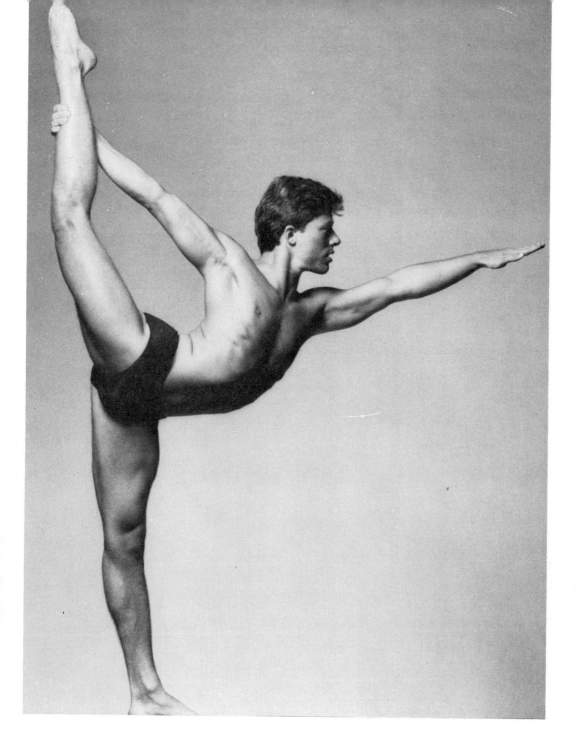

floor and return to Tadasan, taking a full breath. Now repeat the moves on the other side.

Be Aware: Keep chest open and counterbalance the posture with arm in front and leg behind. Keep focused on one point and *breathe evenly*.

Benefits: Keeps back and stomach trim. The deep concentration needed for this pose totally absorbs you into the moment.

Sun Worship

In the Sun Worship, each movement is initiated by either an inhalation or an exhalation.
  (1) Breathe in. Stand in Tadasan with arms out beside body, thumbs and index fingers touching.
  (2) Breathe out, bringing hands to the prayer position.
  (3) Breathe in, stretching arms up into the air, and look up between your fingertips. Now stretch up and bend backward from shoulder blades. Keep seat tight.

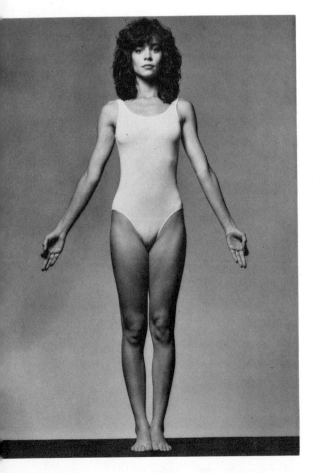
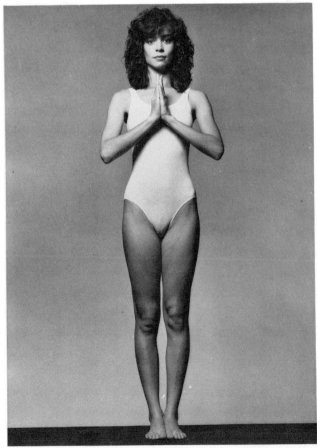

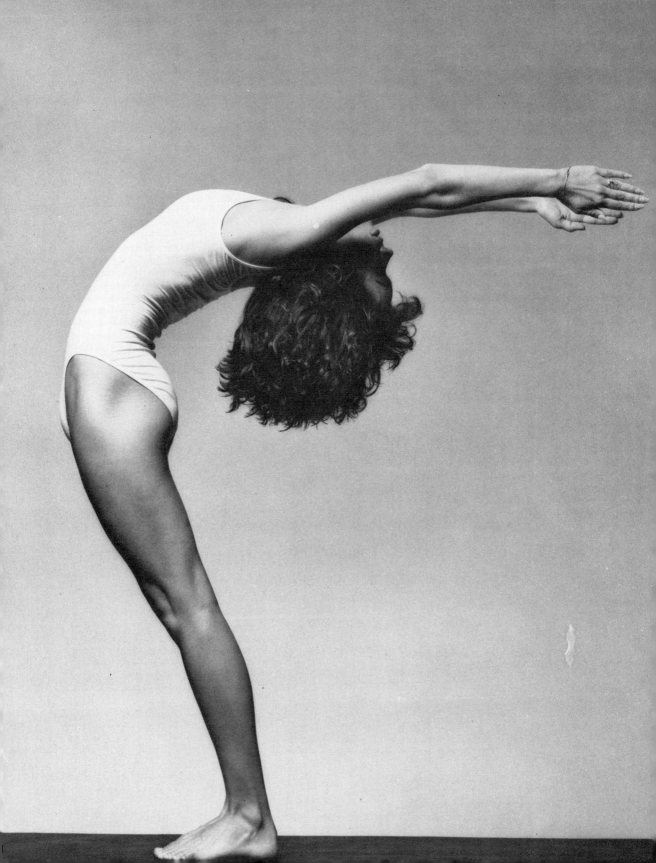

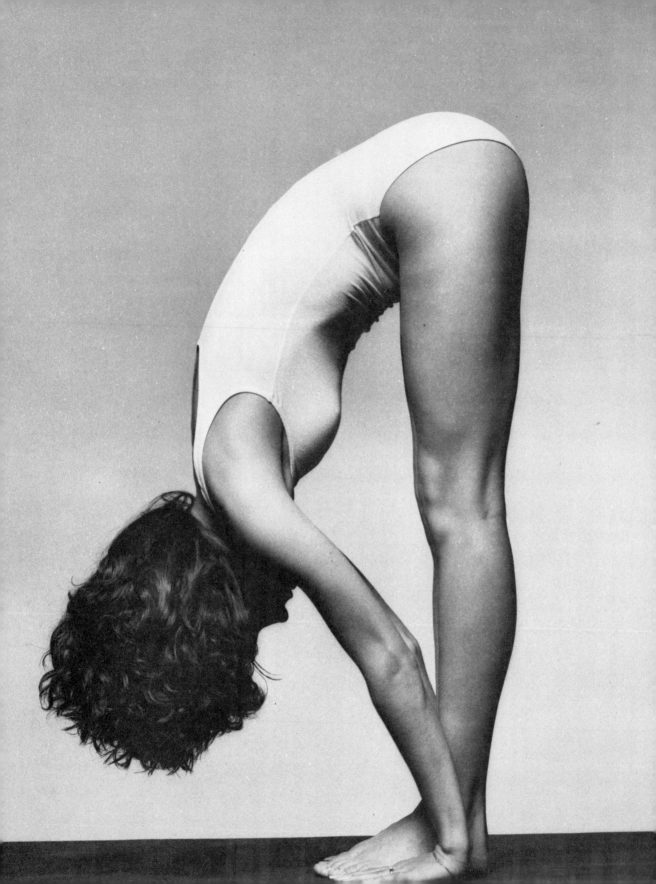

(4) Breathe out and bend forward. Place hands onto the floor beside feet.

(5) Breathe in, bending the right leg and stretching the left leg back as far as possible and as straight as possible. Your face should be lifted toward ceiling, eyes looking down. *Face is relaxed.*

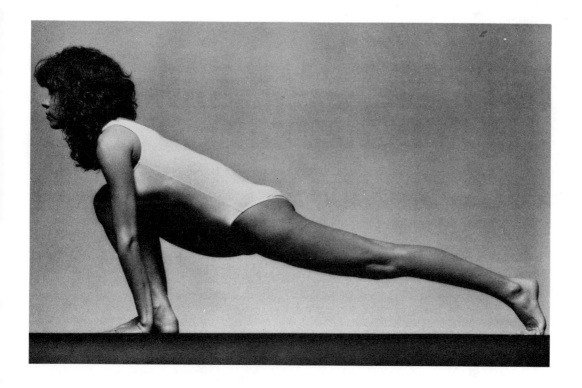

(6) Breathe out and bring right leg back. Stretch both legs and body into a straight line.
(7) Regulate your breath and do a push-up (lower your body to 6 inches off the floor). As you advance and strengthen you can add more push-ups.
(8) Breathe out and lie flat down on the floor.

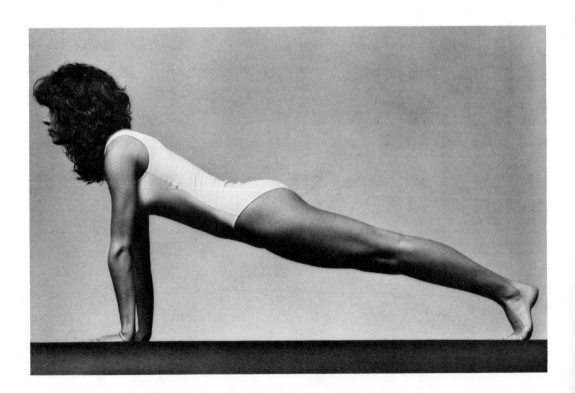

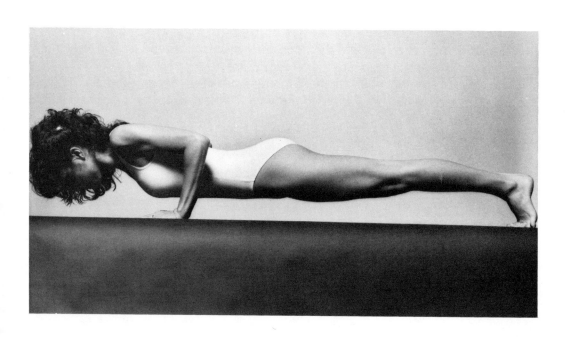

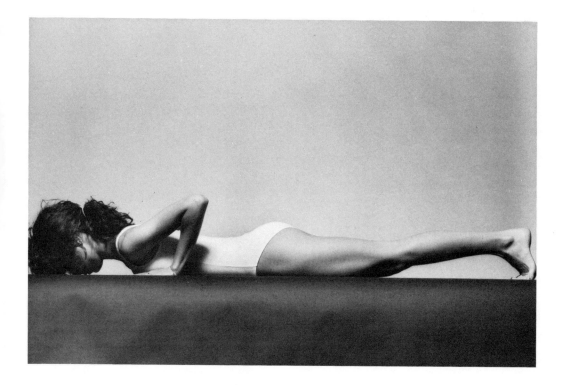

(9) Breathe in, straightening arms and pointing toes. Press body up from the hips into a backbend (the Cobra Pose).

(10) Breathe out, bend toes into the floor, press seat up into the air and straighten legs. Press seat as far up into the air as possible.

(11) Breathe in, pulling your left foot forward between hands. Stretch right leg straight out behind you, knee off the floor. Chest expands and face should be lifted toward the ceiling.

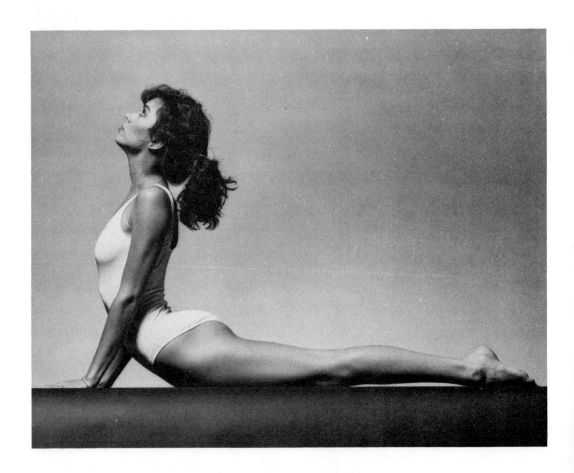

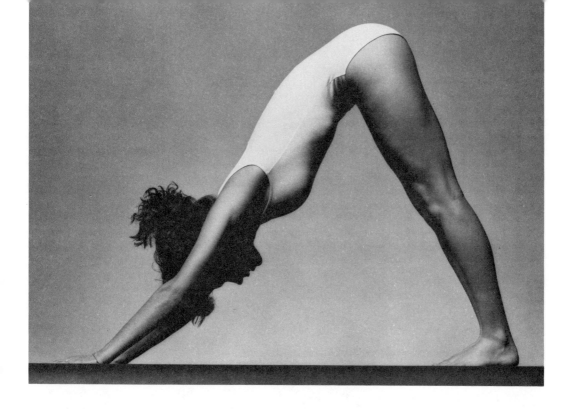

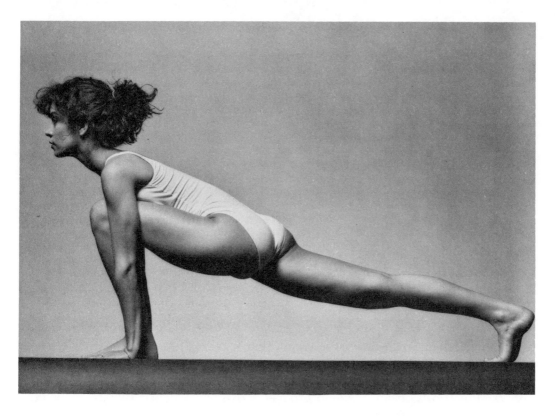

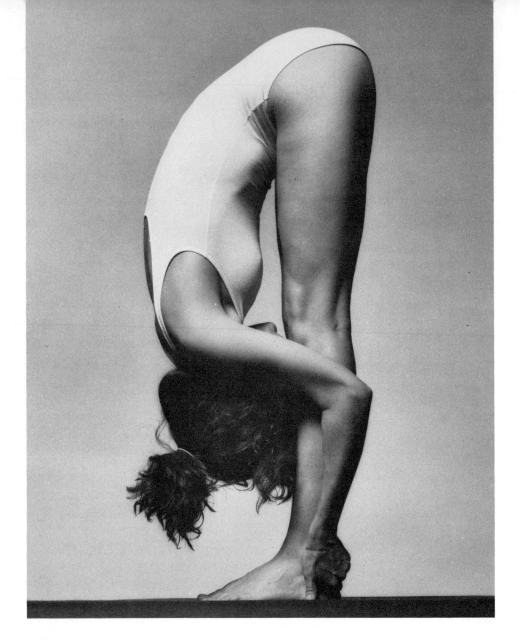

(12) Breathe out and bring right leg forward so both feet are together between hands. Grab heels with your thumbs placed on the floor, keeping elbows bent behind calves. Straighten legs as much as possible, pressing seat up into the air.

(13) Breathe in, come up to a standing position with arms raised toward the ceiling.

(14) Breathe out, drop your arms down beside you to the starting position and into Tadasan. Allow breath to adjust and you are ready to repeat the process.

The Sun Worship can be done as a workout on its own up to 12 times.

Be Aware: Each time you do this your timing will be different. Keep the form in each movement. *The breathing is crucial.*

Benefits: The Sun Worship offers you tremendous cardiovascular therapy, as it puts your body through all the major movements. It gives you the most complete movement range of all the postures.

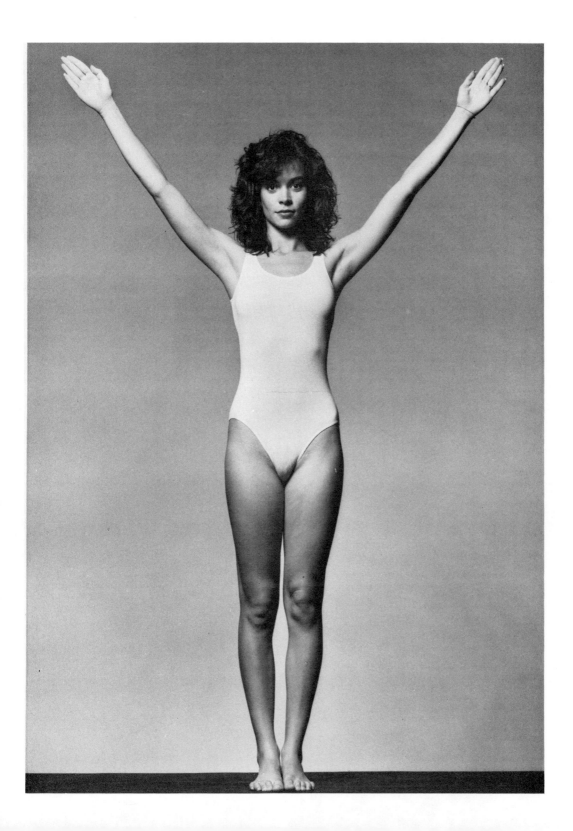

Shoulder Stand

Moves In:

(1) Lie on back with arms down beside you. Bend knees up into the air and continue the movement, rolling up onto shoulders. Placing knees to forehead, support back with palms of your hands. Allow yourself to adjust for 3 breaths.

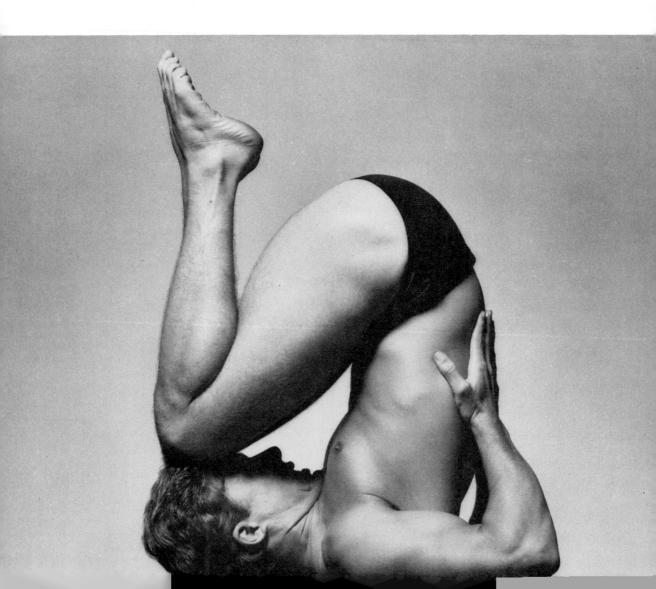

(2) Lift bent knees up into the air with heels dropped to seat. Hold for another 3 breaths.

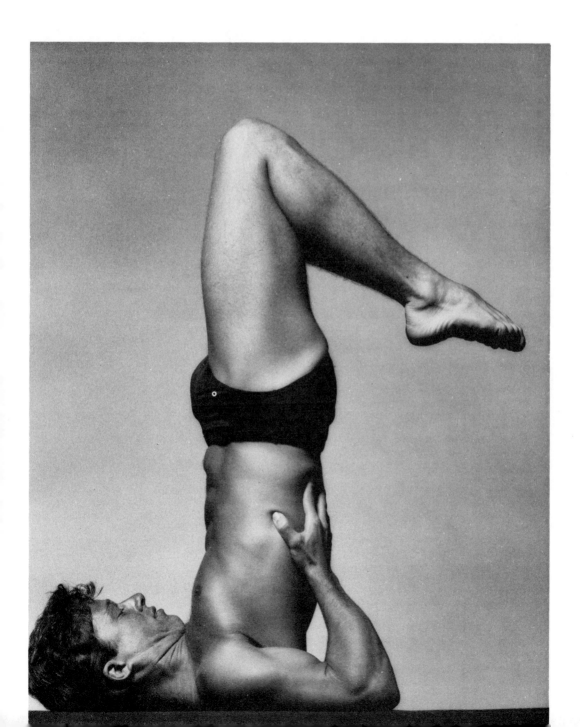

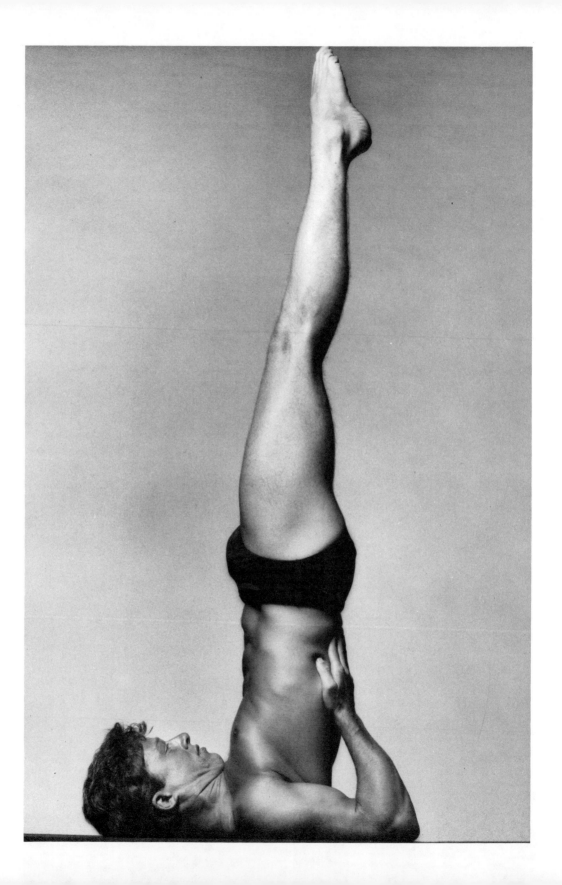

(3) Straighten legs up into the air. Keep weight on elbows, not on neck. Hold the pose, eventually for up to 3 minutes.

Don't move out. Move to Plow Pose below.

Be Aware: Do not put pressure on neck; use seat and stomach muscles.

Benefits: This reverses gravitational pull on your body, totally rejuvenating your body. It is especially good for the thyroid.

Plow

Moves In:

From the shoulder stand lower both feet toward the floor behind your head. Be sure to bend from the hips, not from the spine. Hold for 10 breaths.

Don't move out. Move to Spider Pose on next page.

Be Aware: Keep hips up as high as possible.

Benefits: This gives a tremendous massage to all the organs in the digestive system. Stops constipation.

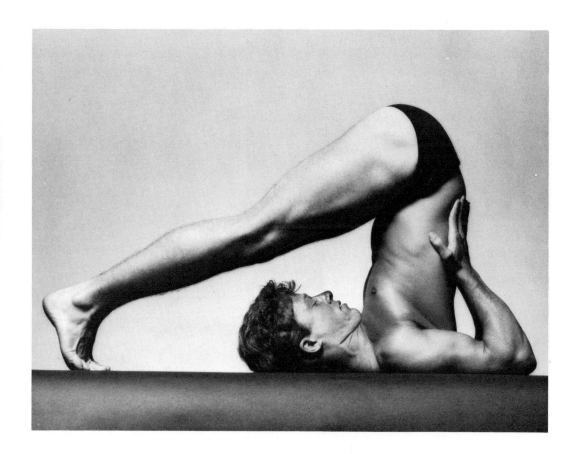

Spider

Moves In:

(1) From the Plow Pose bend knees, placing a knee on either side of your head.

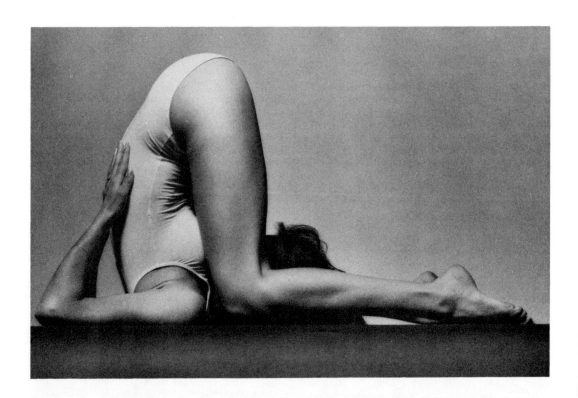

(2) When you can do this comfortably, bring hands over legs and put them under your head. Hold for 30 seconds, breathing slowly.

Moves Out:

Take hands out from under your head and straighten legs out behind head.

Move to Roll Back on next page.

Be Aware: Use stomach muscles and thighs to keep seat bone pressed up in the air.

Benefits: Brings full elasticity to spine. Massages entire digestive system. Creates a radiant appearance.

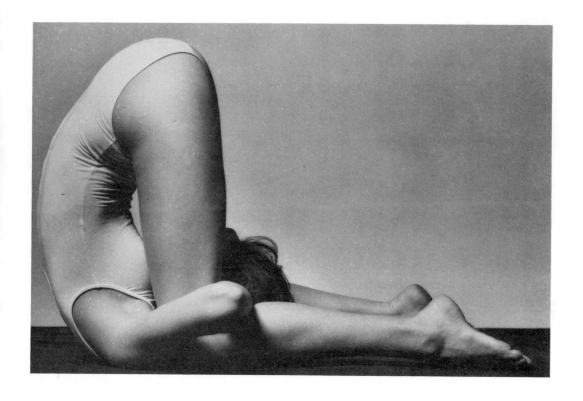

Roll Back

Moves In:

(1) Stretch arms back and grab ankles.

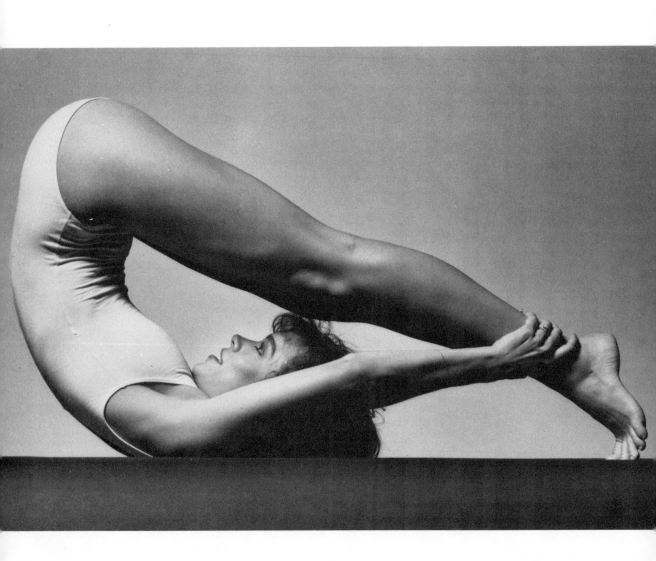

(2) Slowly roll down, vertebra by vertebra, with legs skimming by face. Do not rush; feel spine falling into alignment as you roll down slowly.

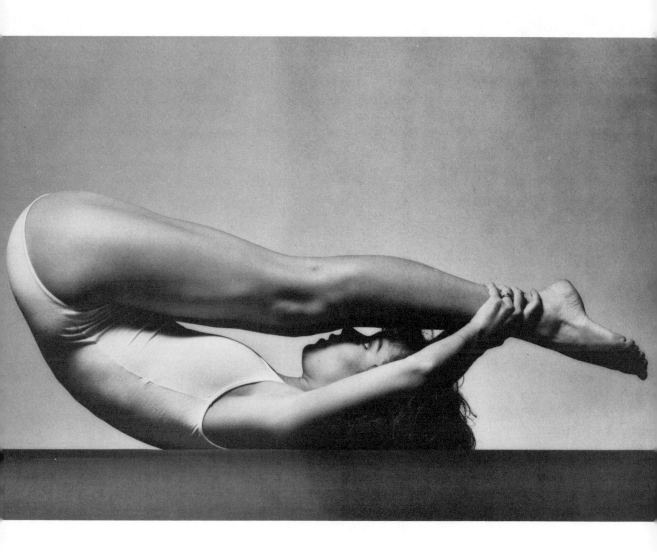

(3) Stop when legs are at right angles to the floor.

Go directly into the Lever, next page.

Be Aware: At first you may need to use your arms to support your back, giving you the control you need to balance.

Benefits: Stretches and aligns the spine, creating a massage of blood around the sensitive nerves in the spine.

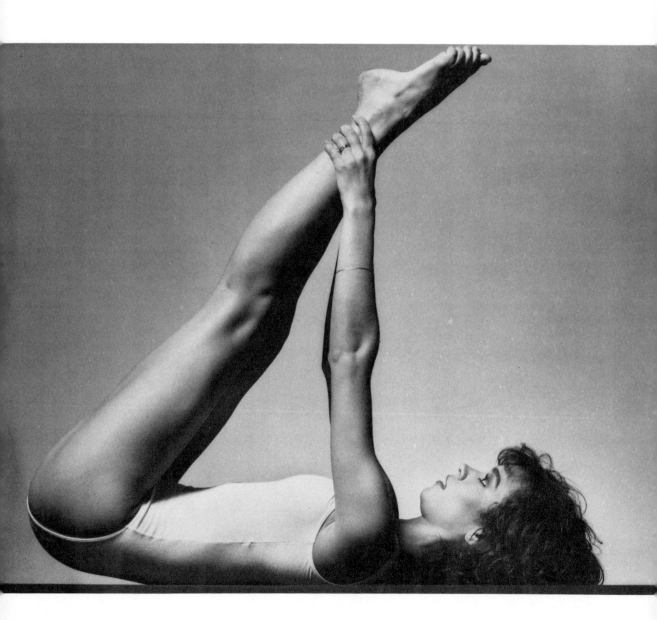

Lever

Moves In:

  (1) Lying on back with legs up in the air, interlace fingers and clasp hands behind head, pulling chin toward chest.

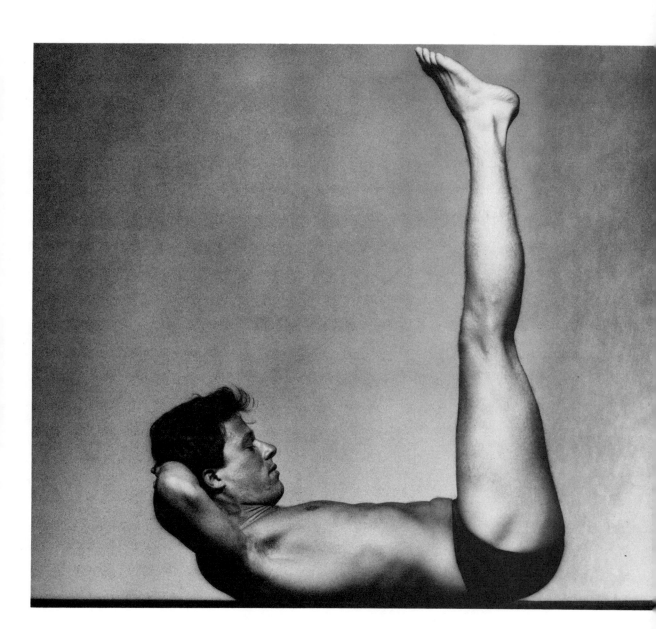

(2) Feeling frontal thighs and stomach muscles tight, flex feet back toward you and lower legs to floor slowly.

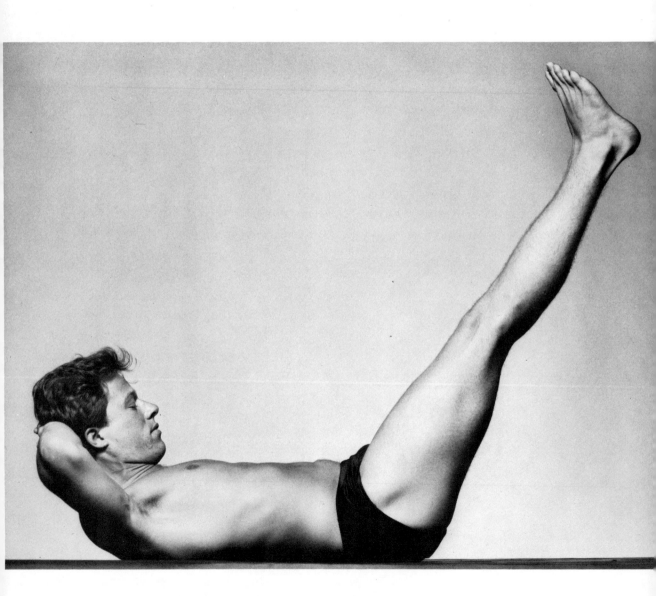

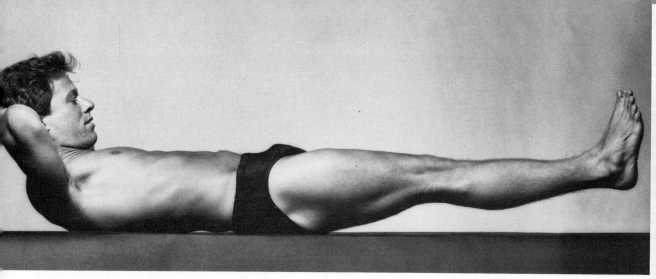

(3) When legs are 6 inches from the floor, hold them there for 3 full breaths, or as many as are comfortable or possible.

Moves Out:

Lower legs and head to floor so your body is flat and relaxed.

Be Aware: Keep spine flat on the floor while lowering and holding legs.

Benefits: Strengthens stomach muscles and keeps spine long; gives one a youthful appearance.

Relaxation-Meditation

Corpse Pose

Lie on your back on the floor, positioning yourself carefully so that each side of your body is equally balanced. Place a cushion under your head or shoulder blades if desired. Turn your attention to your breathing. As you inhale, your stomach rises and you feel the breath move up into your chest. As you exhale your stomach falls and your chest empties.

Continue concentrating on your breathing, watching the rising and falling of your breath, keeping it full and deep without forcing it. Eventually you'll find your breath and your mind becoming still. You will feel a pause between breaths. This pause is a moment between thoughts, a state where you're beyond thoughts. At this moment imagine yourself floating on a cloud, beyond time, space, and form, relaxing and letting go of tension in every part of your body. Remain in this state for a few minutes. If your mind wanders come back to your breath. Follow your breath again to bring yourself back to the feeling of tranquillity.

When you're ready to come out of the relaxation bring your attention to the tip of your nose. Using one nostril at a time, breathe in, trying to visualize blue light in your left nostril. As you breathe out through your right nostril, visualize gold light. Then reverse; gold light as you breathe in right, and blue light as you breathe out left. Slowly stretch out and bring your attention back to a waking state.

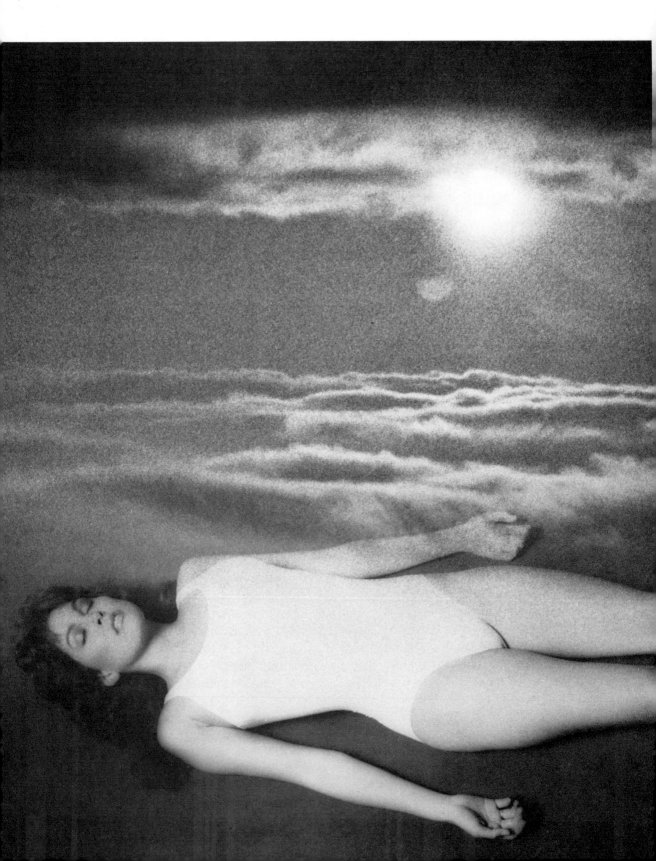

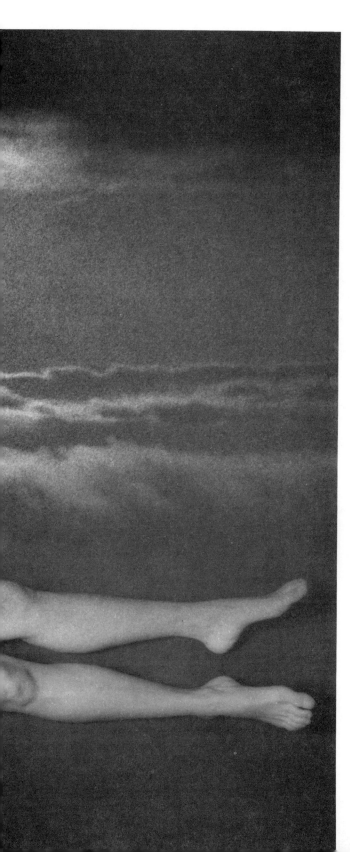

We must begin to open up the communication channels of awareness within our bodies. If you pay regular attention to your body, then scanning it for signs of strain or tension in this relaxation exercise will feel familiar. You may discover through this exercise that your internal environment is just as accessible as your external one. By tensing, flexing, relaxing and moving each bodily part you will recognize—often for the first time—the many shades of experience that lie within you. Take your time to explore sensations you may never have consciously observed before.

Like any new endeavor this exercise will become more self-healing with practice.

It is advisable for you to make a cassette recording of this technique and play it back, reading slowly and allowing time to carry out every move.

Moves In:

(1) Lie on your back to get body balanced and comfortable. Place a cushion under your head if you're uncomfortable.

(2) Take a full breath in. Lift left leg up into the air approximately 6 inches off the floor. Tighten all the muscles in your left leg. Breathe out and relax the leg, placing it back on the floor. Feel a healing warmth in the leg. Repeat with other leg.

(3) Take a full breath in. Pull left arm up into the air approximately 6 inches off the floor, make a fist and tighten arm. Breathe out, place the arm back down on the floor and feel a warm healing feeling in the arm. Repeat with other arm.

(4) Roll head from one side to the other slowly, then center head and feel a warm healing feeling.

(5) Take a full breath in, pinch seat tight together, breathe out, relax seat, and get a warm healing feeling in hip structure, genital area and arms.

(6) Take a full breath in and blow the abdomen up. As you breathe out feel abdomen fall in and get the warm healing feeling in the abdomen area.

(7) Take a full breath in, fill chest, then breathe out and relax chest, feeling that warm feeling in the rib cage.

(8) Take a full breath in and tighten facial muscles. As you breathe out relax face and feel a warm healing in face.

(9) Now feel the whole body warm and healing, each cell recharging.

(10) Having balanced and healed the body, we come to heal the mind. As you breathe out feel that you exhale any and all thoughts. Continue this until no thoughts are left. Again, you'll experience a state beyond thoughts, a state of freedom, of non-doing, of inner silence, of inner peace. Enjoy this state for 5 to 10 minutes.

Moves Out:

(1) Run thumbs over fingertips, and wriggle toes to get energy back to your extremities.

(2) Stretch arms and legs out. Now you're ready to face life again.

Be Aware: Don't let your mind's restless nature distract you. Hang in with the technique; the mind will quiet. Keep your mind your servant and companion, not your master.

Benefits: Total relaxation and physical, mental and spiritual healing.

Hand to Big Toe

Moves In:

(1) Lying on back, bend right leg up into the air and with the right middle finger, index finger and thumb, grab hold of right big toe. Place left hand on left thigh and hold it down on the floor.

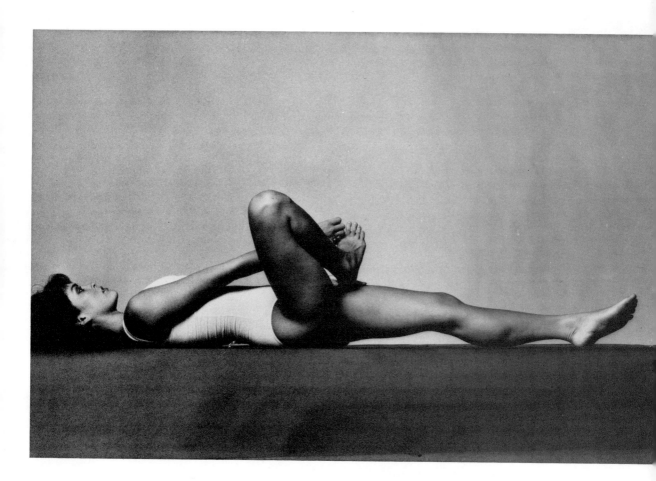

(2) Straighten right leg up into the air as far as you can, your right elbow turned outward. Hold for 5 breaths.

(3) Pull leg to forehead, lifting head off floor. Breathe evenly for 6 breaths.

(4) If you can't reach foot, a towel will help. Place the towel over the arch of your foot and hold the ends in either hand. Eventually you will stretch out those muscles and tendons.

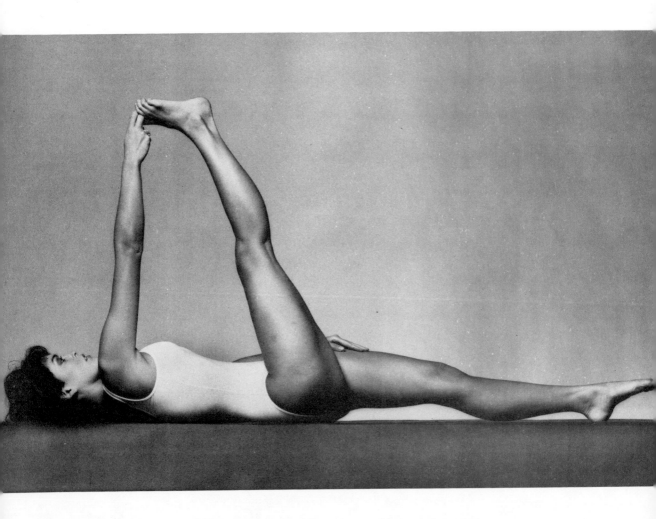

Moves Out:

> Place head back on the floor and release the right leg down to the floor. Take a full breath. Repeat on other side.

Be Aware: Keep the stretch from the seat bone to the heel. Tightening your thighs will help.

Repeat posture on other side.

Benefits: This pose releases tension from the hamstrings. Yogis believe that it's in the hamstrings that we hamper unconscious emotions. It also releases pressure from the spine, giving a sense of being energized.

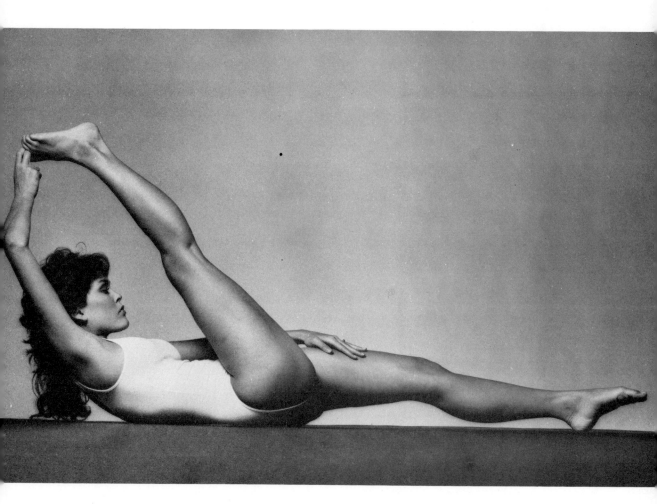

Scale

Moves In:
  (1) Sitting on the floor, bend knees up and catch hands behind them.

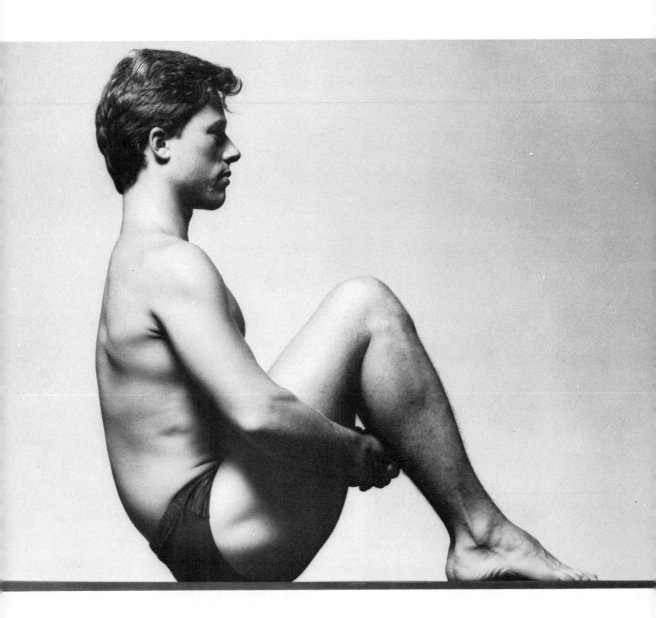

(2) Balance on seat bone, remembering to keep spine straight. Take a full breath in and on the exhalation lift legs up into the air, straightening them.

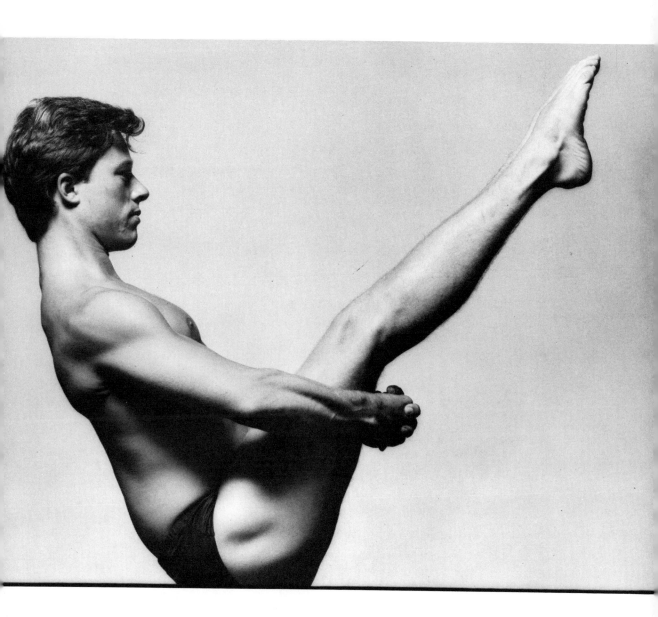

(3) When your balance is secure, stretch arms out toward legs, *parallel to the floor.* Hold the pose for 6 breaths or 15 seconds.

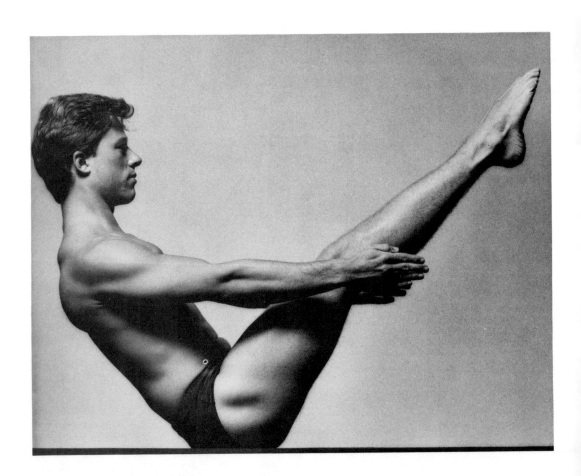

(4) If you've mastered the pose, interlace hands behind head. Keep spine tall and toes at eye level. Hold the posture for 15 seconds more.

Moves Out:

Clasp hands behind knees and bend knees, placing feet back on the floor. Place hands on knees and take a full breath in *through the nose and out through the lips.*

Be Aware: Don't bend the spine in order to balance. Keep chest expanded. Tighten the front of thighs. Press heels forward.

Benefits: Firms stomach, seat and thighs. Strengthens heart muscles and increases circulation.

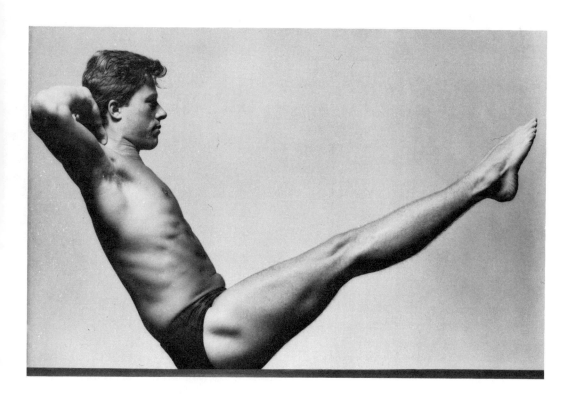

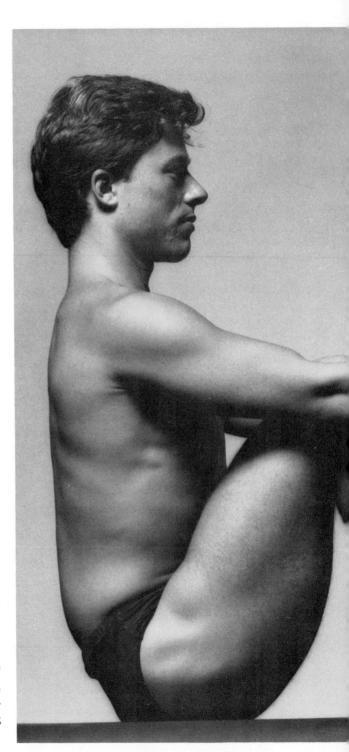

Scale with Partner

Moves In:

(1) Both partners sit on the floor facing each other, knees bent and toes touching. Clasp each other's wrists.

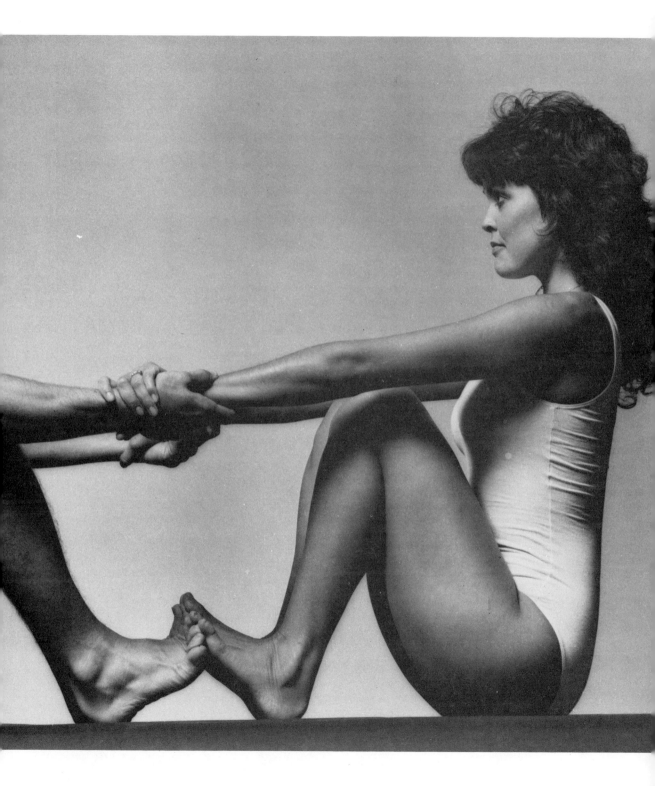

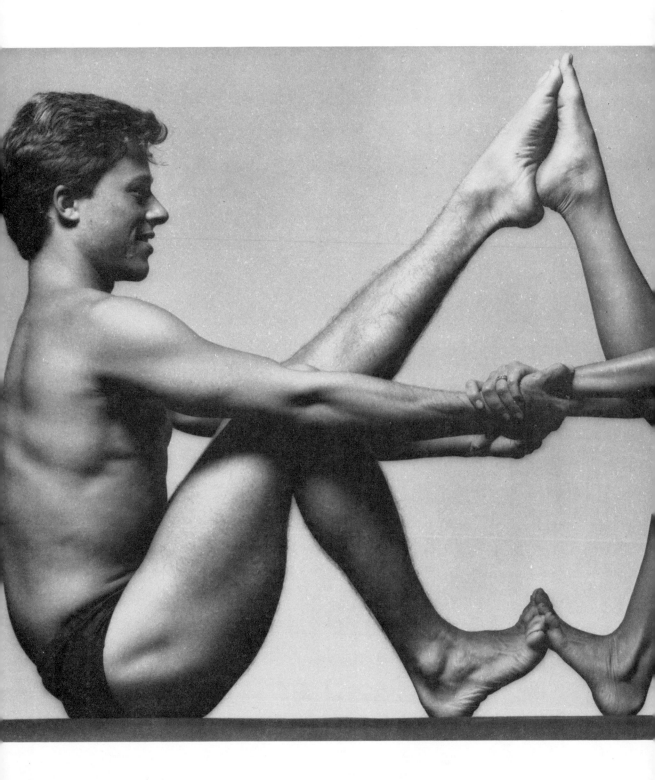

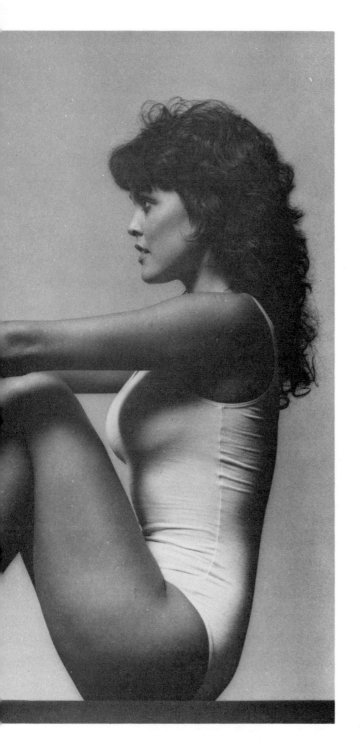

(2) Pushing against each other's feet, press first one leg then the other up into the air.

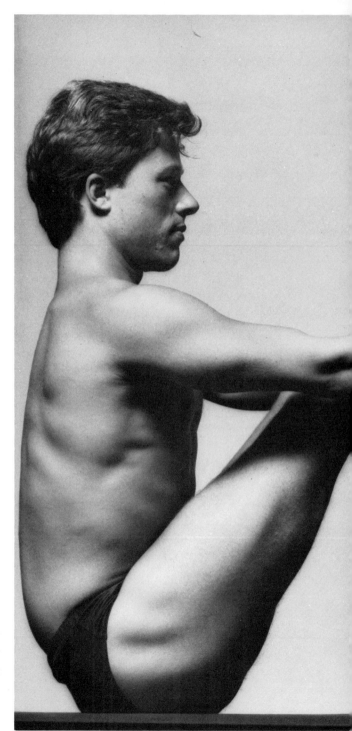

(3) Pulling against each other, get spine straight.

Moves Out:

(1) Lower one leg down at a time.

(2) Place hands on knees and take a full breath in through the nose and out through the mouth.

Be Aware: Keep balanced on seat bone. Keep feeling the spine straight.

Benefits: This pose dramatically improves your posture: that is, it keeps you tall, it strengthens the stomach, thighs and seat muscles. Improves breathing.

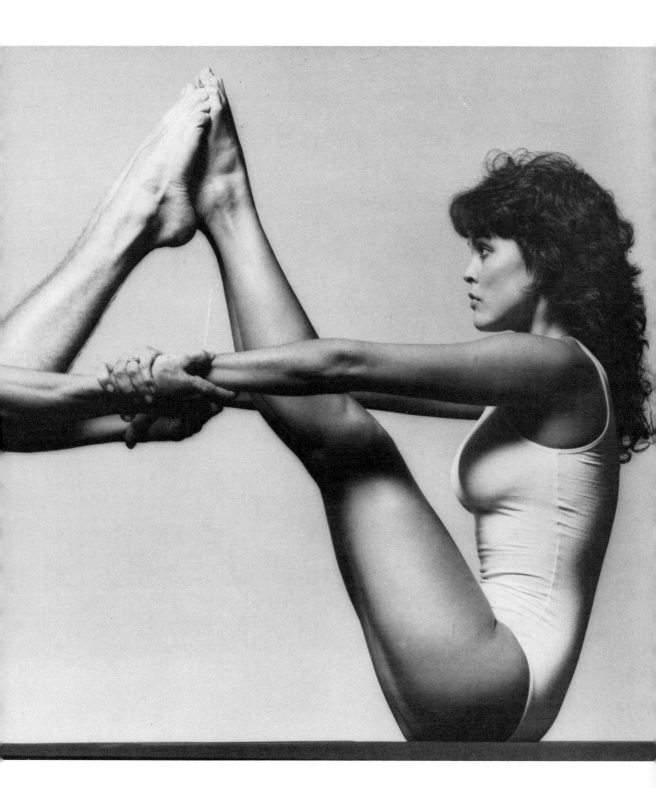

Bow

Moves In:

(1) Lying on stomach on the floor, bend knees and grab ankles from the outside.

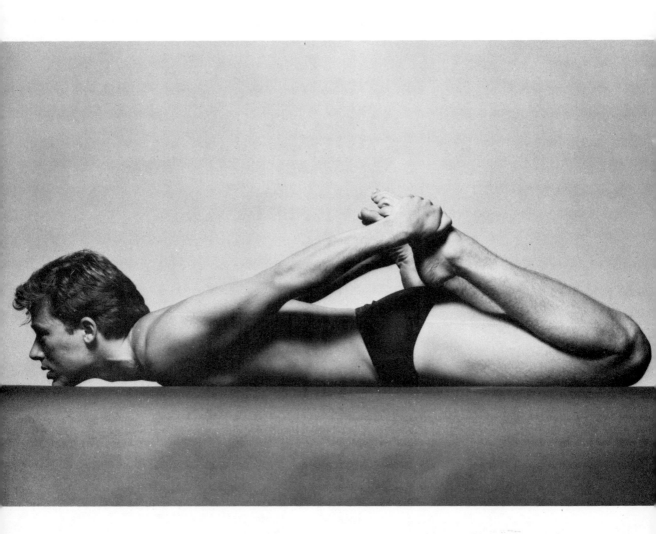

(2) Lift chin, neck and chest up off the floor.

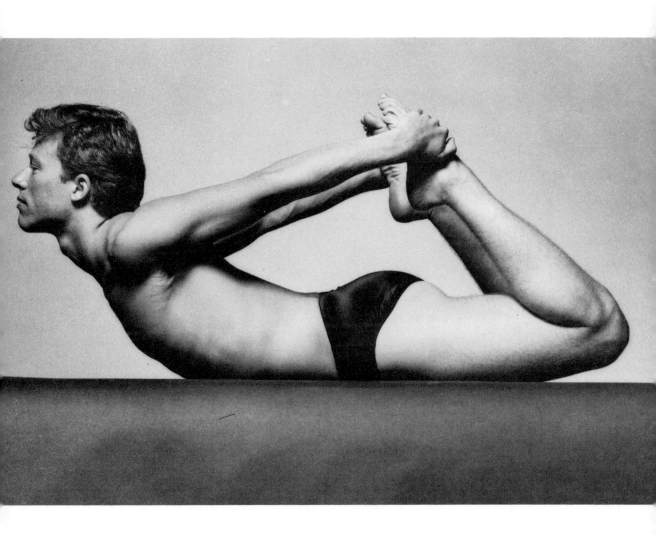

(3) Then lift legs, pushing feet higher and higher up and over body. Breathe for 10 breaths.

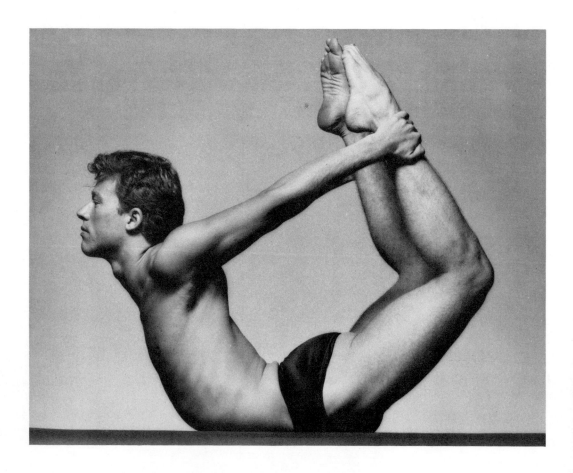

(4) Lower the torso and legs slowly. Let go of feet and lower them to the floor; put arms on the floor beside you.

Moves Out:

Turn head to one side and relax, then to the other side and relax.

Be Aware: Do not strain in the pose if you have high blood pressure. Release pressure from lower back by stretching legs back and torso forward. Keep chest expanded and face relaxed with eyes looking downward at a 45-degree angle.

Benefits: Revitalizes spinal nerves, stops slouching, improves digestion, strengthens and firms abdominal muscles, thighs and arms.

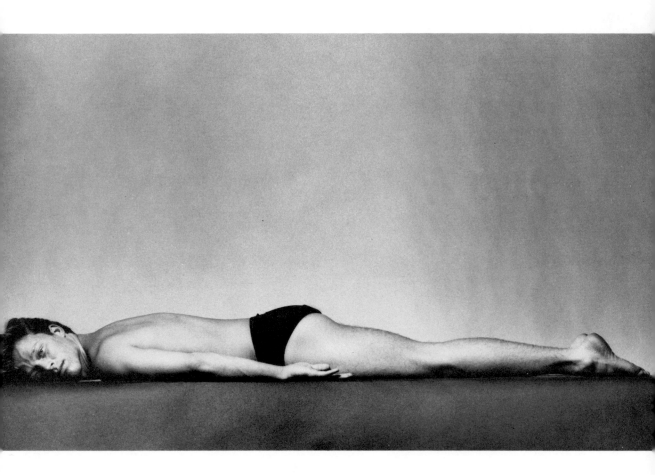

Tent

Moves In:

(1) Kneel on all fours on the floor, about 4 inches of space between the feet, the hands and the knees, and curl toes into the floor.

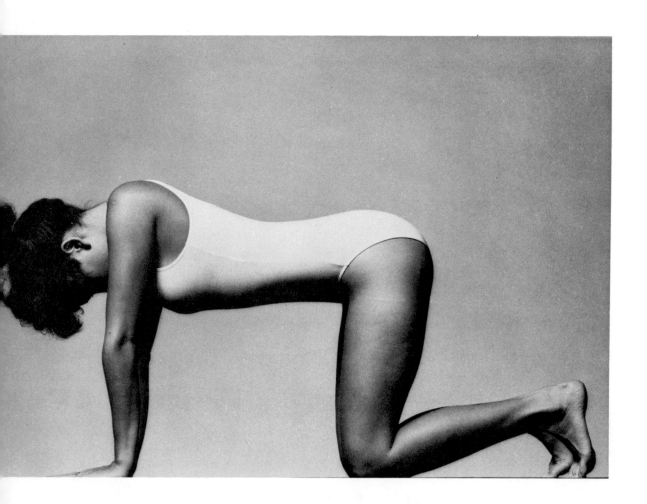

(2) Straighten legs and come up on toes, seat bone up into the air and head toward the floor, feeling spine stretching long. Hold for 6 breaths.

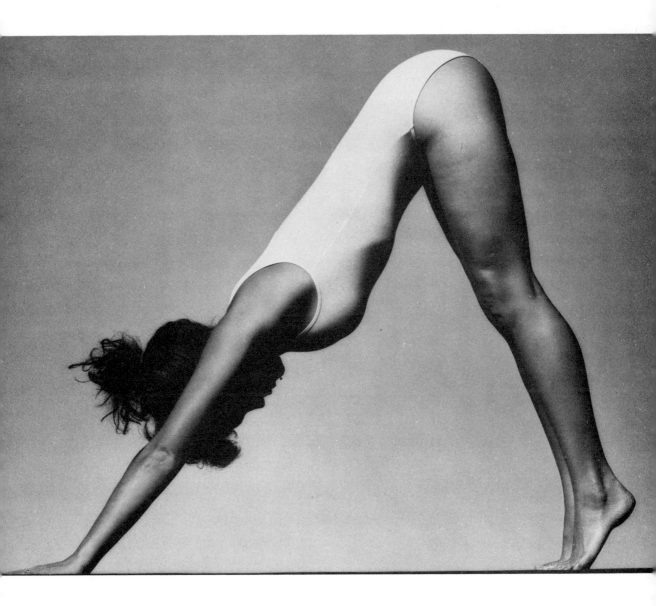

(3) Drop the soles of feet onto the floor but keep pressing seat bone up into the air and legs straight. Hold for 6 breaths.

Moves Out:

Bend knees and slowly lower them to the floor. Point toes out behind you and sit back onto heels (Japanese style), placing hands on thighs. Take a full breath in through your nose and out through your mouth.

Be Aware: Your frontal thighs should be tight. Keep pressing seat bone up into the air.

Benefits: Stretches entire back of body from Achilles' tendon up your legs, down your back, shoulders, and arms. Improves breathing as it opens the chest.

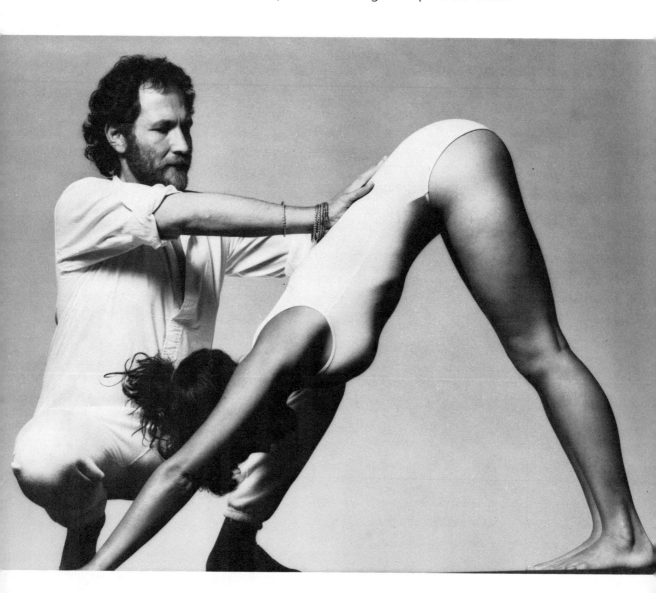

Tent with Partner

Moves In:

(1) Kneel on all fours and hold the ankles of your partner, who stands in front of you with feet parallel about one foot apart.

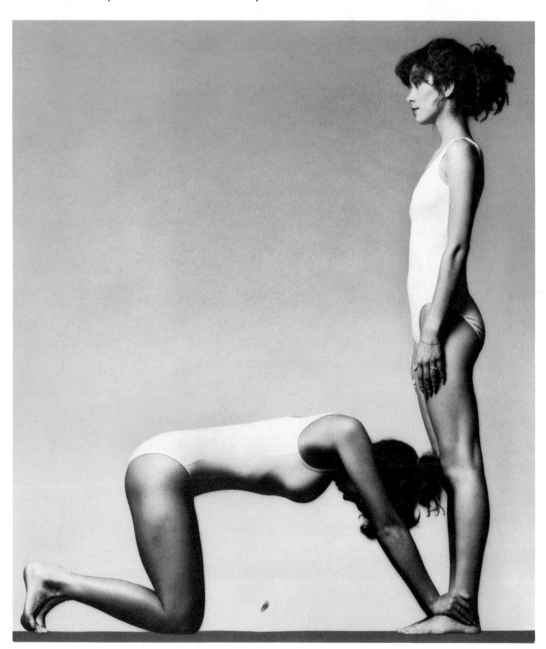

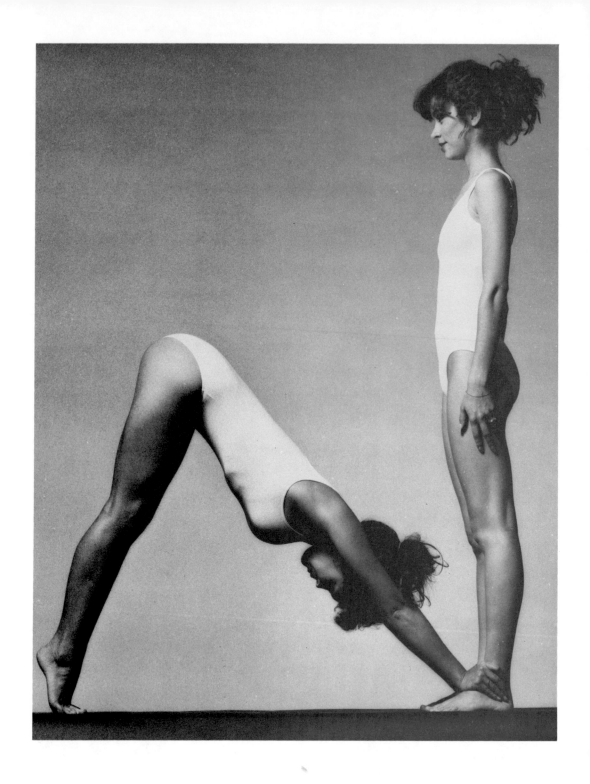

(2) Straighten your legs, pressing seat up into the air.

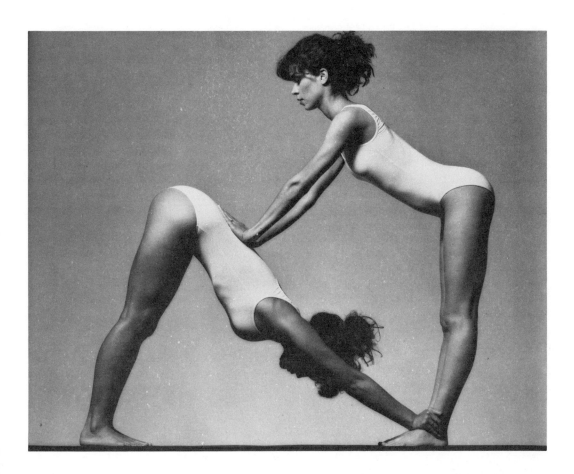

(3) Then place feet flat on the floor. The standing partner places hands on the small of your back and presses your spine so that it flattens. Hold for half a minute to a minute.

Moves Out:

(1) Bend your knees to kneel down on the floor.
(2) Sit back on your heels and take a full breath in through your nose, and out through your lips.

Be Aware: Hold your standing partner's ankles, not feet.

Benefits: The same as the Tent, except one gets added leverage from the partner.

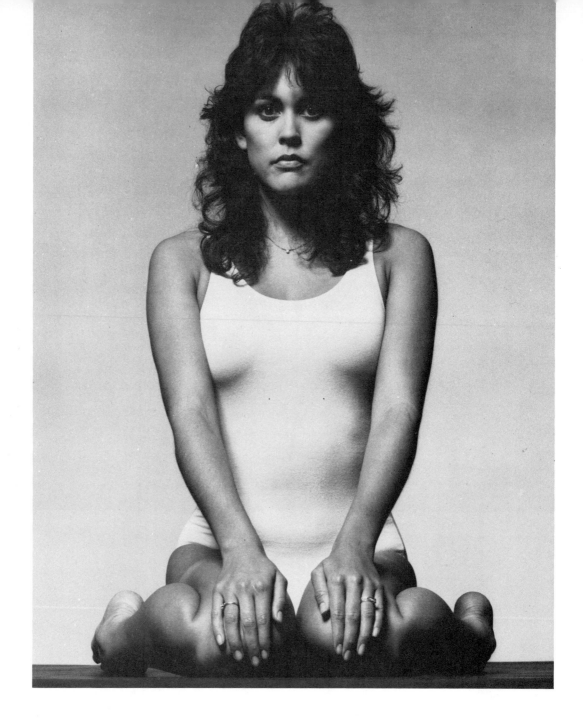

Fish Twist

Moves In:
(1) Sitting on heels (see Diamond Seat, page 125) keep knees together, open feet apart and keep big toes and little toes on the floor. Sit on the floor between feet.

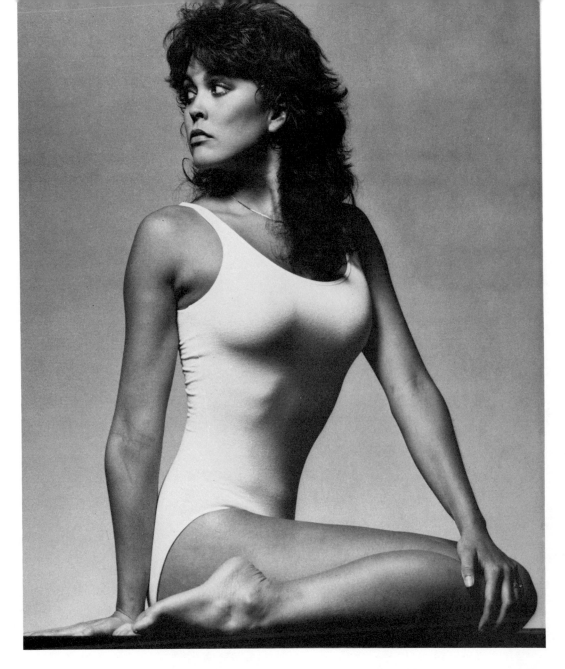

(2) Place left hand on right knee and right hand on the floor behind you. Look over right shoulder, face relaxed, and hold for 3 breaths. Reverse and do the other side.

Moves Out:
 (1) Return to center.
 (2) Take 3 full breaths.

Be Aware: Keep your spine tall and straight, then rotate around it.

Benefits: Loosens hips, relieving pressure on sciatic nerve. Massages liver, spleen and colon. Keeps bowel movements regular.

Fish I

Moves In:

(1) Sitting on heels (see Diamond Seat, page 125), keep knees together, open feet apart and keep big toes and little toes on the floor. Sit on the floor between feet.

(2) Holding sole of foot with hand, bend one elbow to the floor.

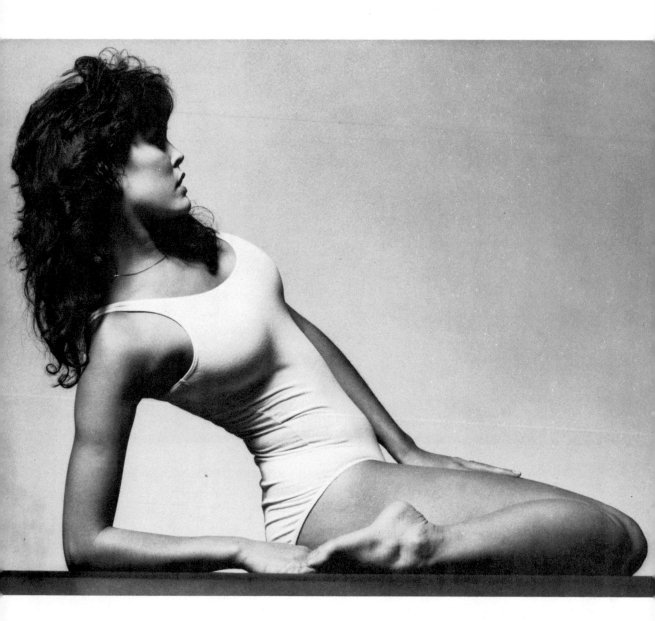

(3) Bend the other elbow onto the floor behind you so that your torso is leaning back supported by arms.

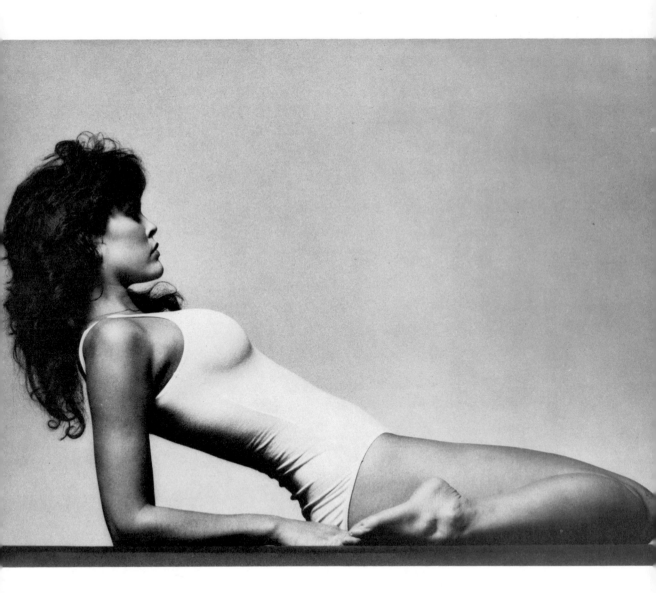

(4) Slowly place head on the floor.

(5) Now, extend arms on the floor behind head. Hold for 10 breaths.

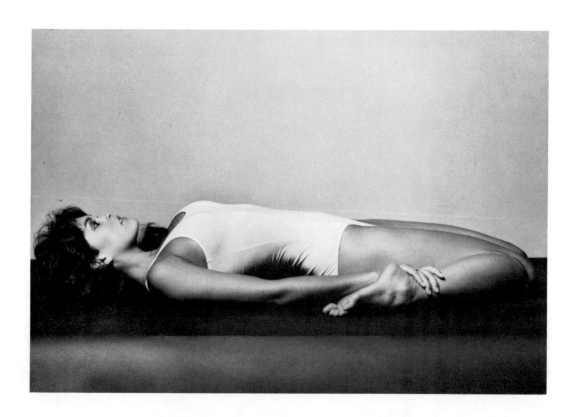

Moves Out:
 (1) Hold ankles, use elbows and then hands to come up slowly.
 (2) Looking forward, take a full breath in through the nose and out through the mouth.

Be Aware: Don't strain knees or lower back. Use the muscles around shoulder blades to lift chest, avoiding too much pressure on neck. There should be no pain in knees.

Benefits: Stops rheumatism, improves breathing, and heals breathing ailments.

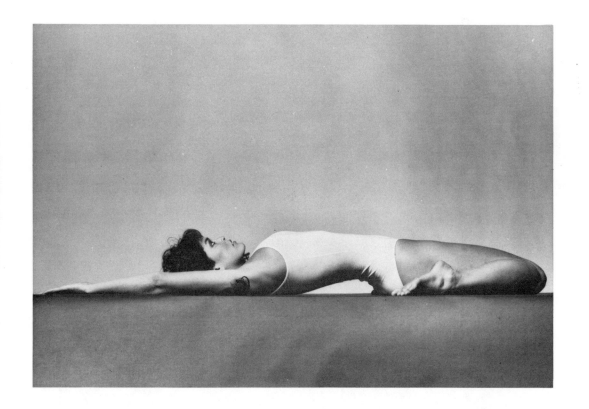

Moves In:

   (1) Sitting between feet, place hands on the soles of feet.

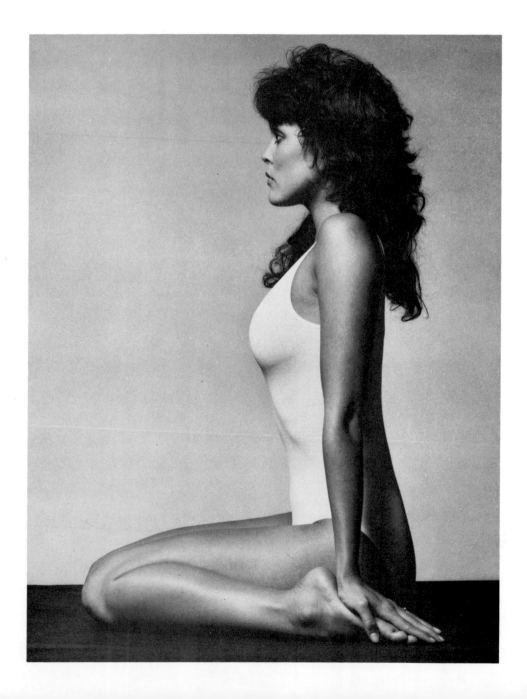

(2) Take a full breath in and then exhale. Move forward to place head on the floor in front of knees. Pull seat back down onto floor. Hold this posture, building up to 10 breaths.

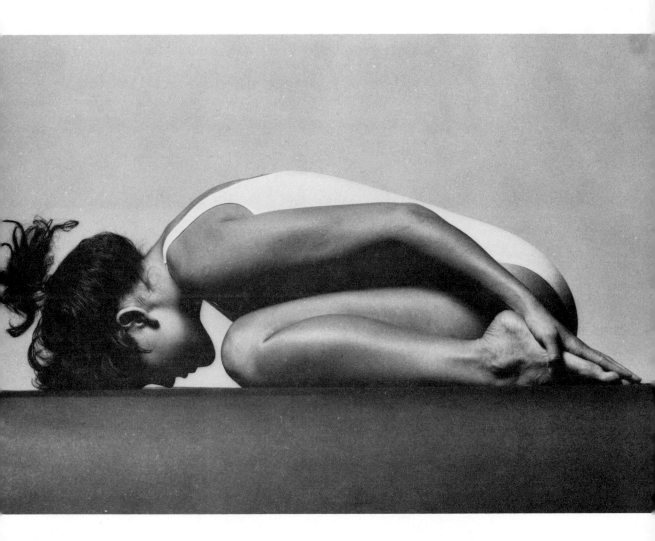

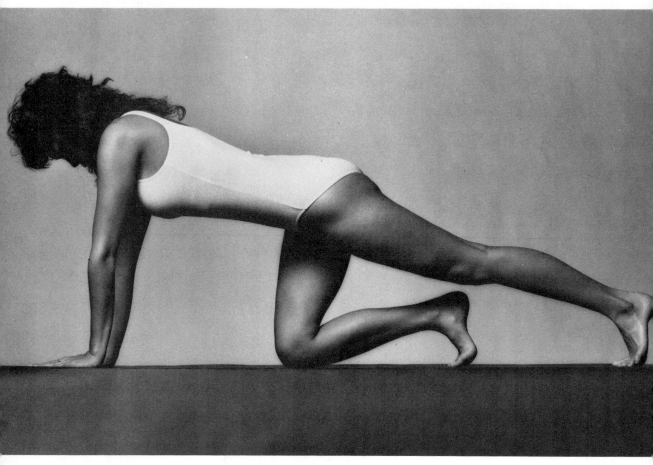

Moves Out:

(1) Pull yourself up to sit tall. Place hands on knees. Take a full breath in through your nose and out through your mouth.

(2) Kneel onto all fours and stretch one leg straight back behind you. Then change legs.

(3) Sit back onto heels (see Diamond Seat, page 125). Take a full breath in through your nose and out through your mouth.

Be Aware: Stretch spine long, relax neck and face. Breathe evenly.

Benefits: Unlocks tension from hips, gives your spine its correct alignment and nourishes the nerves and organs in the hip and sacrum region.

Camel

Moves In:

(1) Kneel with lower legs out behind you. Place the palms of hands on your lower back.

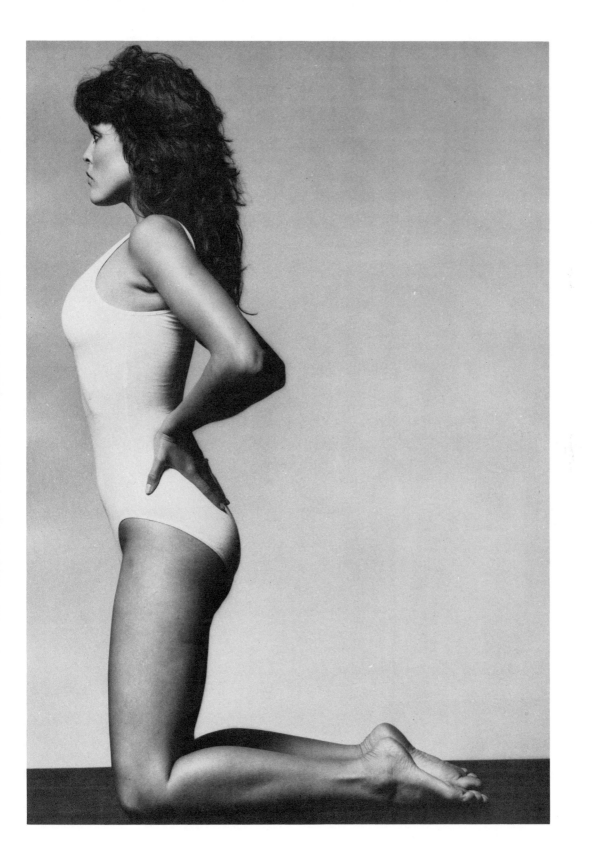

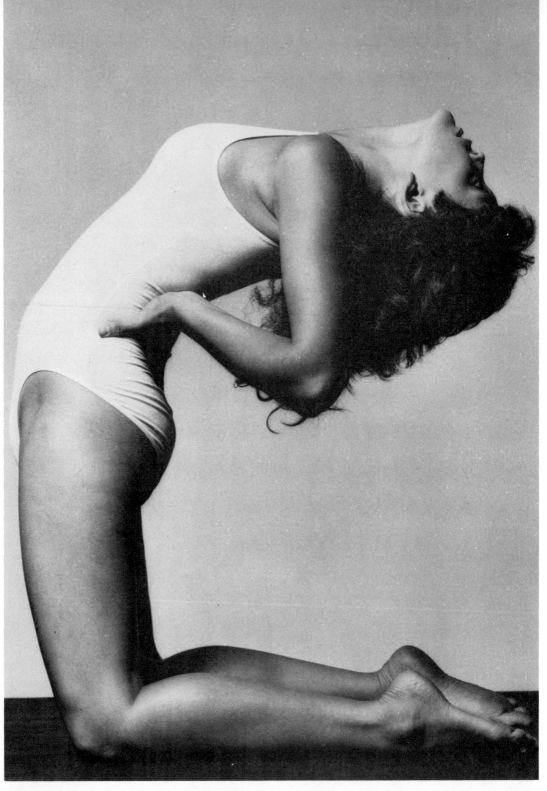

(2) Take a full breath into stomach, let the air expand into chest, and relax the head back.

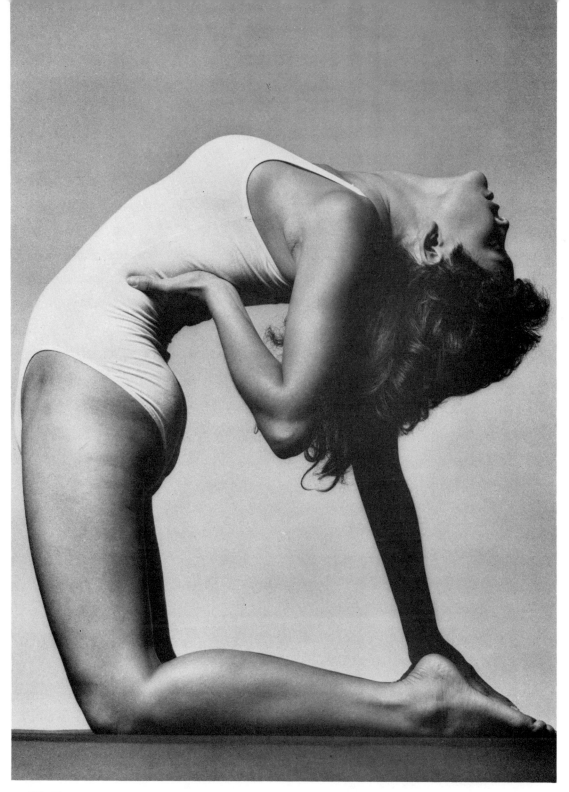

(3) Tighten seat. Breathing out, bend back around shoulder blades to place one hand at a time on the soles of feet.

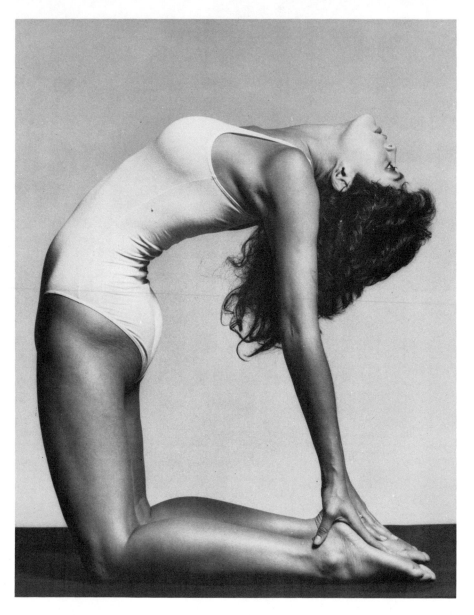

(4) Keep seat tight and press thighs forward. Breathe through, holding the pose for up to 10 breaths.

Moves Out:
Bring one hand up to lower back to give it support, then the other. Tighten seat muscles and pull yourself to come up tall, still kneeling, keeping chin stretched back to let blood pressure readjust. Then lift head to upright position and breathe smoothly.

Be Aware: Use the muscles of seat and frontal thighs to project spine up, and bend backwards around shoulder blade.

Benefits: This pose creates tremendous flexibility in the spine, sending nourishment to the spinal column and your nervous system. It also massages the digestive system and trims the waistline.

Diamond Seat

Moves In:

(1) Sitting on heels (Diamond Seat) draw arms up into the air, palms together and biceps beside ears.

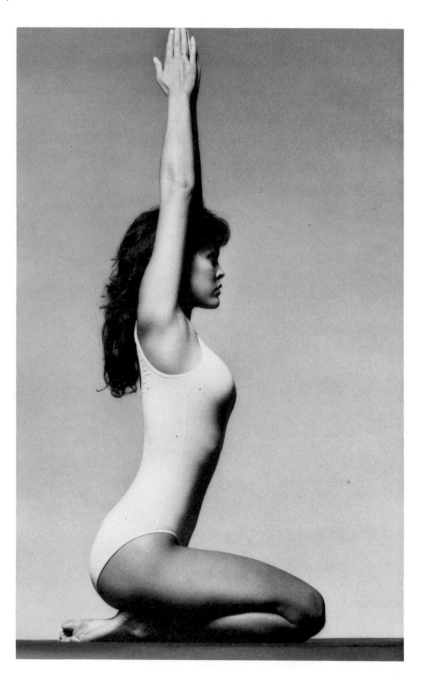

(2) Take a deep breath in and on the exhalation bend forward from the hips, placing the outstretched arms on the floor as far in front of you as possible. Place forehead on the floor in front of knees. Breathe smoothly through for 15 breaths.

Moves Out:

(1) Bring head up so that ears are between the biceps. Take a full breath in and pull yourself up to sit up tall, keeping biceps beside ears.

(2) Drop hands down onto knees, take a full breath in through your nose and out through your mouth.

Be Aware: Use stomach muscles to move into and out of the pose. Keep seat on heels.

Benefits: This offers tremendous traction to the spine, relieving spinal problems.

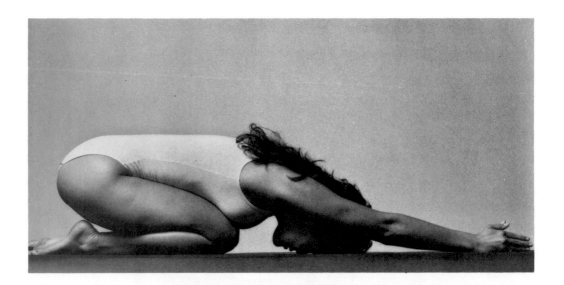

Cat

Moves In:

(1) Kneel onto all fours, knees hip-distance apart, hands on the floor directly under shoulders. Breathe in, tilt hips up and stomach down, raise face to look up.

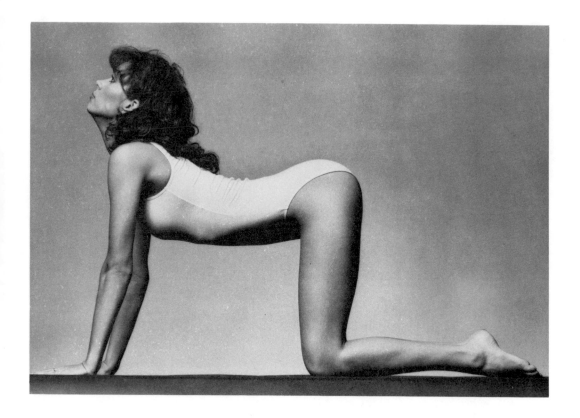

(2) On the exhalation hump back up, release hips down, lower chin into chest and pull stomach in.

Repeat 3 times.

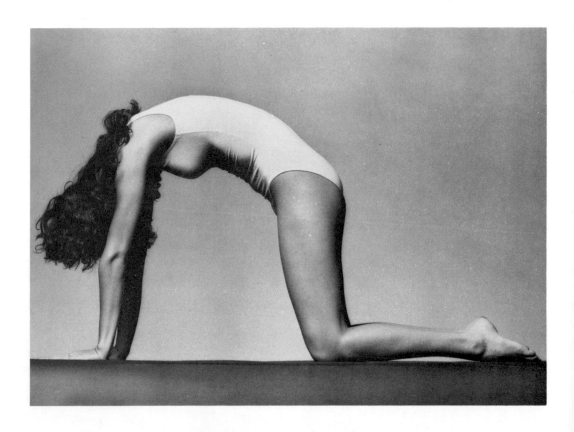

(3) Rotate the hips (moving them to the side, down, to other side, and up), creating a large circular movement with the spine.

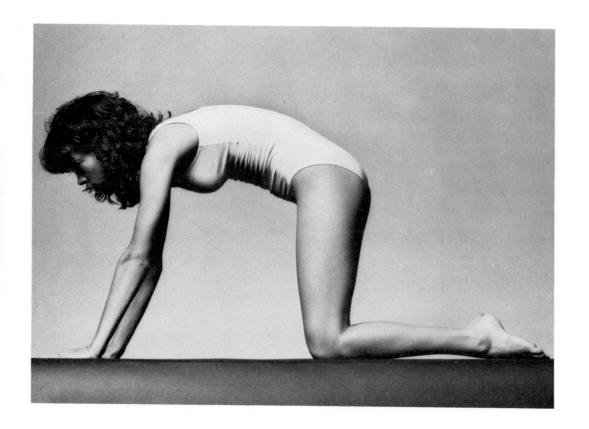

(4) Do 3 times to the left and then reverse, 3 times to the right.

Moves Out:

Lie on your back on the floor.

Be Aware: Keep the movement of spine initiated from hip structure.

Benefits: Massages and rejuvenates spinal column, the central cord of your nervous system.

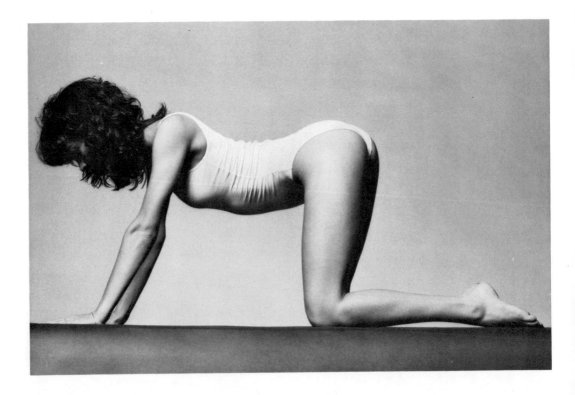

Bridge I

Moves In:

(1) Lie flat on back, bend knees up, feet hip-distance apart, arms down beside you.

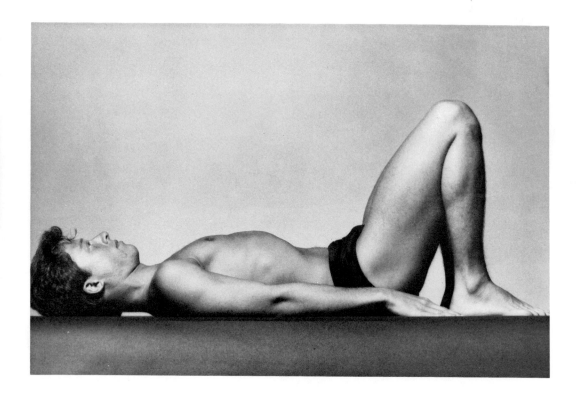

(2) Press seat up into the air, getting thighs parallel to the floor. Feel shoulder blades opening. Hold for 5 breaths.

Moves Out:

Lower back down onto the floor and stretch legs out in front of you. Take a full breath in through your nose and out through your mouth.

Be Aware: Use seat and thigh muscles to press up. Feel the shoulder-blade area opening.

Benefits: Strengthens and shapes thighs, stomach and seat. Releases tension from spine. Stops slouching.

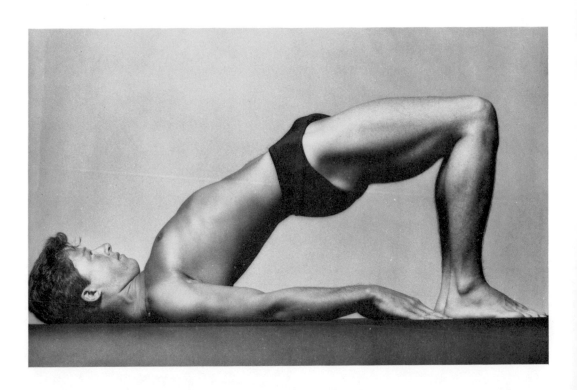

Bridge II

Moves In:
(1) Do the two steps in Bridge I position.
(2) Place the palms of hands on the floor beside ears, with fingers pointing toward feet.

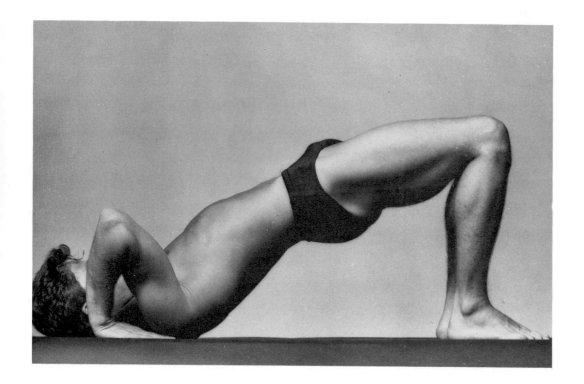

(3) Press on arms, bringing head back so the crown touches the floor.

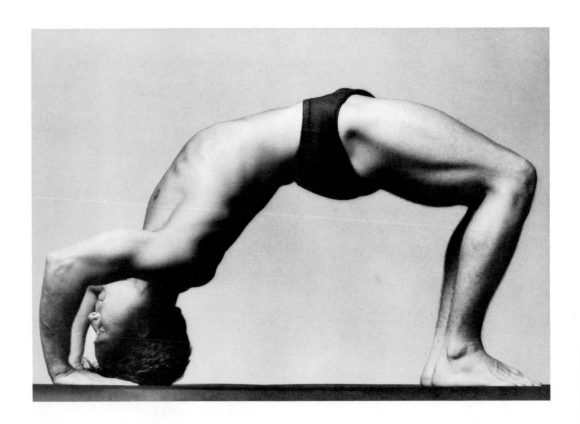

(4) Straighten arms, pushing your whole body up into the air. Keep neck relaxed. Hold for 6 breaths.

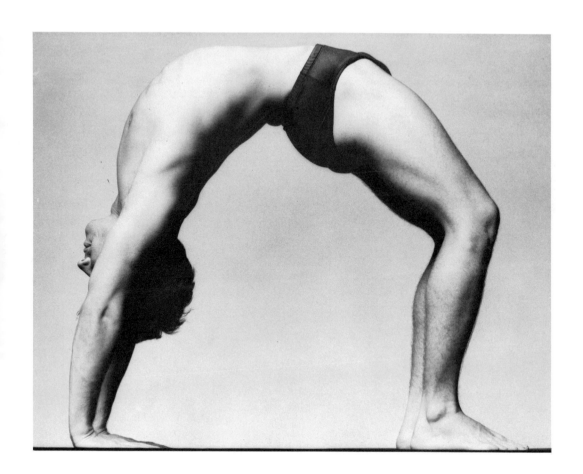

(5) If secure in the pose, walk legs out straight and bring feet together. This offers a greater stretch to the lumbar spine area.

Moves Out:

(1) Walk the legs back in toward body (if you managed to straighten).
(2) Slowly bend elbows, lowering head to the floor.
(3) Take head out from under you and lower your back down to the floor.
(4) Stretch legs out and take a full breath in through your nose and out through your mouth.

Be Aware: Stretch the abdominal wall long, as this causes the lumbar vertebrae to stretch apart. Without this stretch they will be compressed, and pinch on spinal nerves.

Benefits: Strengthens and firms arms, abdomen, lower back, seat and thighs; stretches and realigns spine, massaging the spinal nerves and ligaments. Excellent to cure digestive problems.

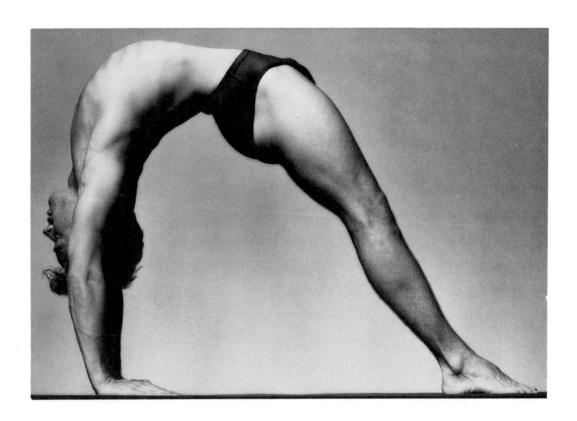

Sparrow

Moves In:

(1) Lie on back. Bend knees up into air and pull the thighs toward abdomen. Interlace fingers and clasp them around the shin bone two inches below the knees.

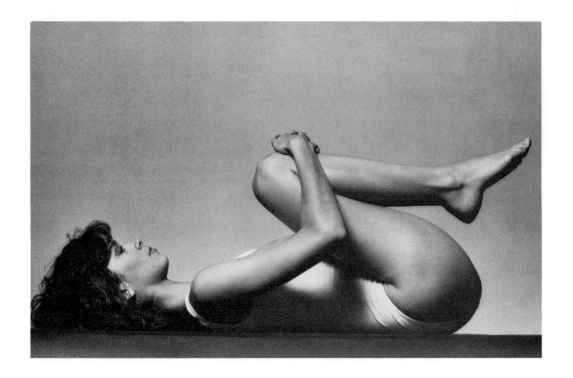

(2) Pull forehead up to knees and breathe smoothly through for 8 breaths.

Moves Out:

Relax head back down onto the floor, then straighten legs out on the floor in front of you.

Be Aware: As you place the head back on the floor, feel the back and neck flattening toward the floor.

Benefits: Massages the digestive organs, releasing gases; realigns hips and spine; stops lower-back pain.

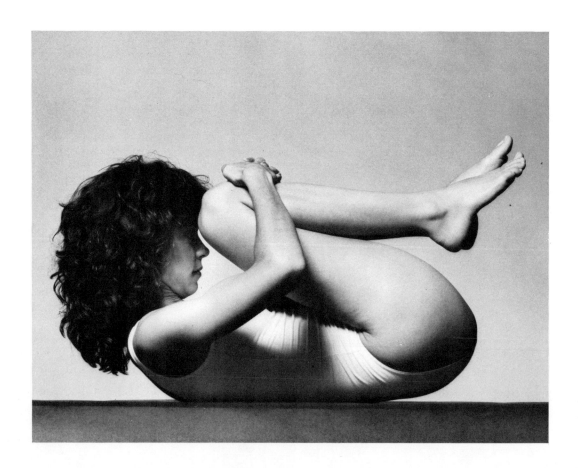

Sit-up

Moves In:

(1) Lying on your back, stretch arms out behind head, the palms together and biceps beside ears. Flex feet toward you.

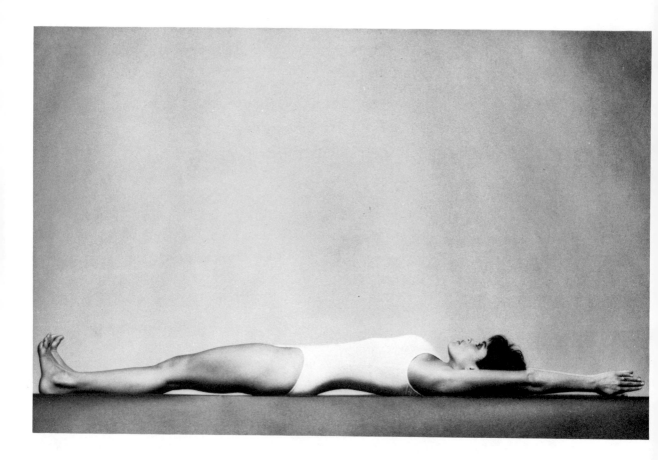

(2) Breathe in. As you exhale pull yourself to sit up tall, trying to keep the biceps beside ears. Use stomach muscles.

Moves Out:

Lower arms down to your sides, take a full breath in through nose and out through mouth.

Be Aware: Try to keep arms beside head. Use stomach muscles and frontal thighs to sit up.

Benefits: Strengthens stomach muscles.

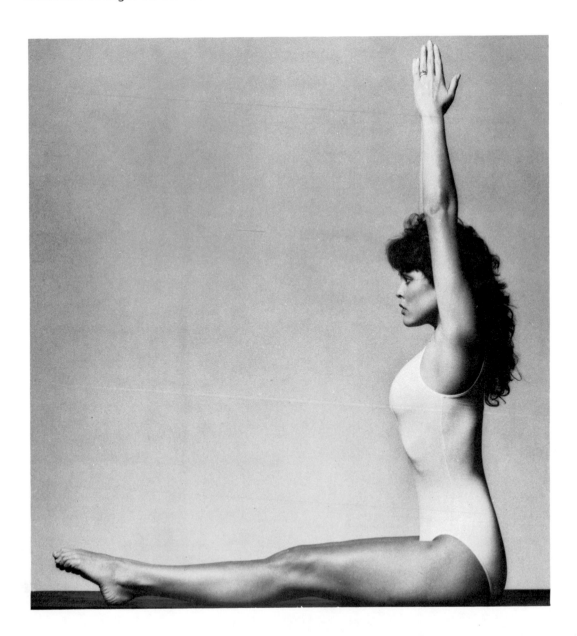

Forward Bend

Moves In:

(1) Sit on floor, with legs stretched out in front of you. Use hands to separate the buttocks.

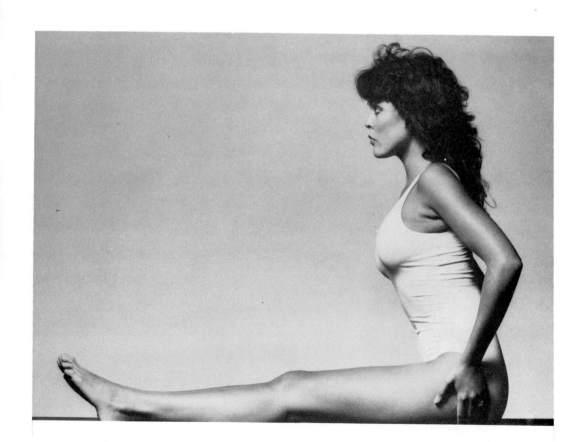

(2) Bend knees and clasp each big toe with index, middle fingers, and thumbs.

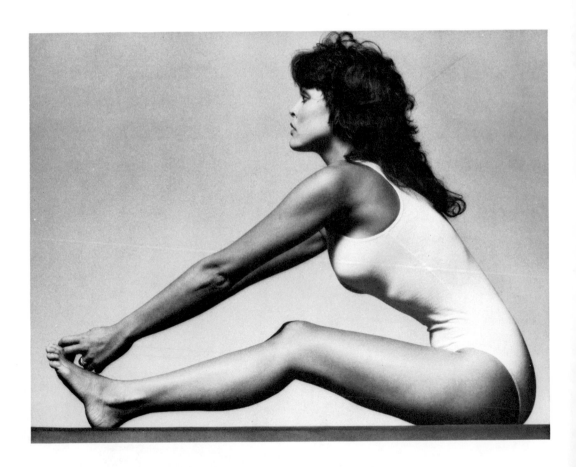

(3) Straighten legs, keeping spine straight and bending forward from the hips.

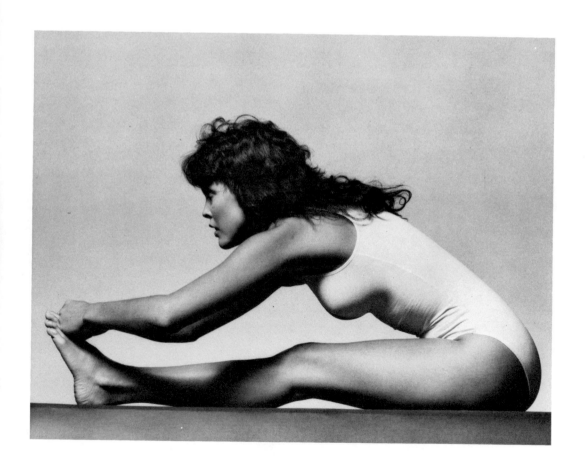

(4) Bend elbows, pulling torso forward over the legs, first the abdomen, then the chest, then the forehead. Hold for 10 breaths.

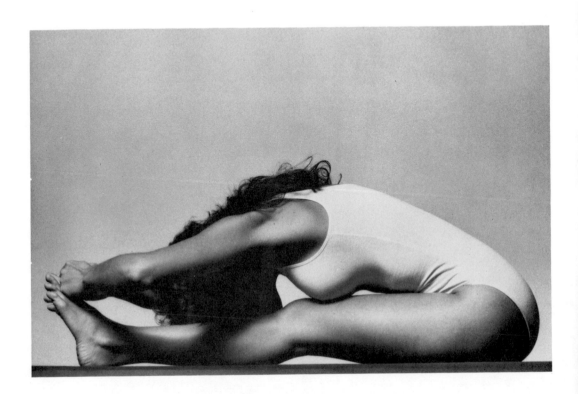

Moves Out:

(1) Breathe in and, still holding toes, lift head, chest, and stomach up, keeping spine straight. Take 3 complete breaths, in through nose, out through mouth.

(2) Breathe out and sit up straight. Place the hands on the floor beside you and let breath adjust.

Be Aware: Don't bend spine in order to get head down. Reach forward from hips. Tighten frontal thighs. Press heels forward and seat bone backward.

Benefits: Creates flexibility in hamstring muscles and sciatic region. Tones bowel, bladder, kidneys and pancreas. Releases pressure from lumbar vertebrae of spine. Releases tension.

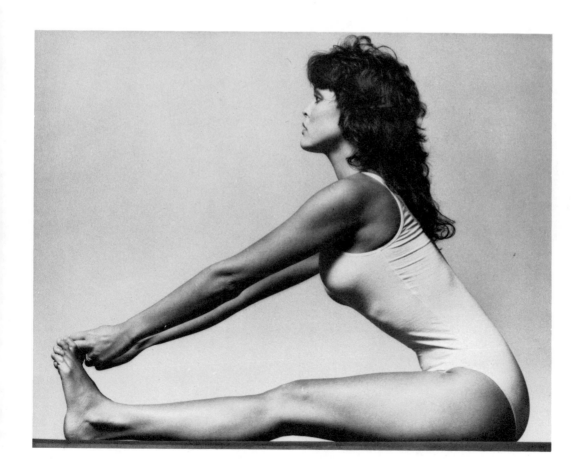

Moves In:

(1) Sit on the floor with legs spread wide apart. Remain seated firmly on seat bone with spine tall. Stretch arms out to the side, parallel to the floor.

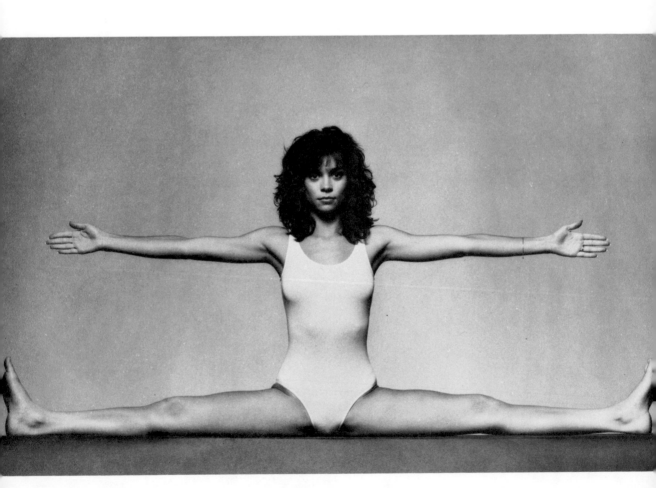

(2) Breathe in and on the exhalation stretch out to the left side, reaching with the left hand to clasp as low down the left leg as possible, eventually clasping the left ball of the foot on the big-toe side. Bring right arm up into the air. Lower it over to the left side, without twisting the torso.

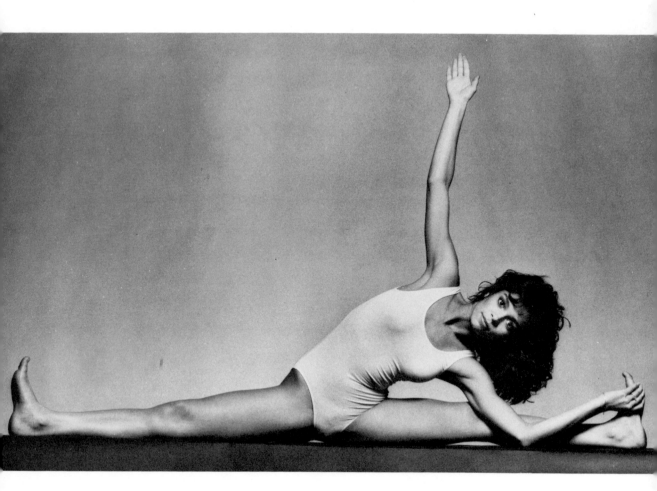

(3) The right hand eventually clasps the left foot from the little-toe side.

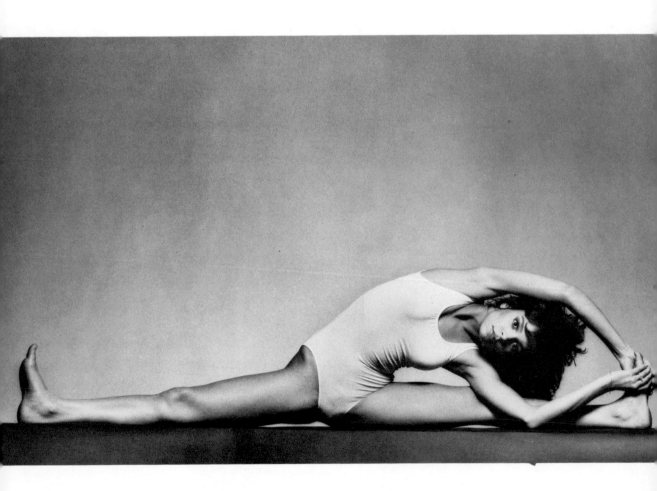

(4) Turn your head to look up toward the ceiling and hold for 5 even breaths.

Moves Out:

Raise the right arm, then the left; sit up in starting position and repeat on other side.

Be Aware: Keep spine stretching out to the side without bending forward into yourself. Keep chest open.

Benefits: Massages the kidneys, keeps the bowel and bladder massaged. Releases tension from spine and hips.

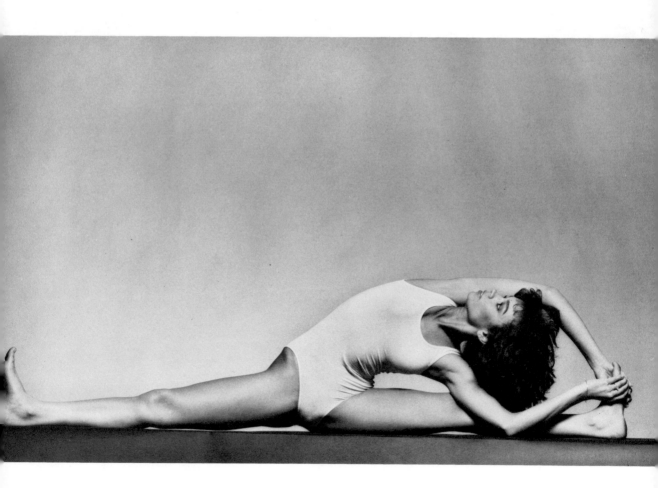

Moves In:

(1) Sit on floor with spine tall and legs spread wide apart.

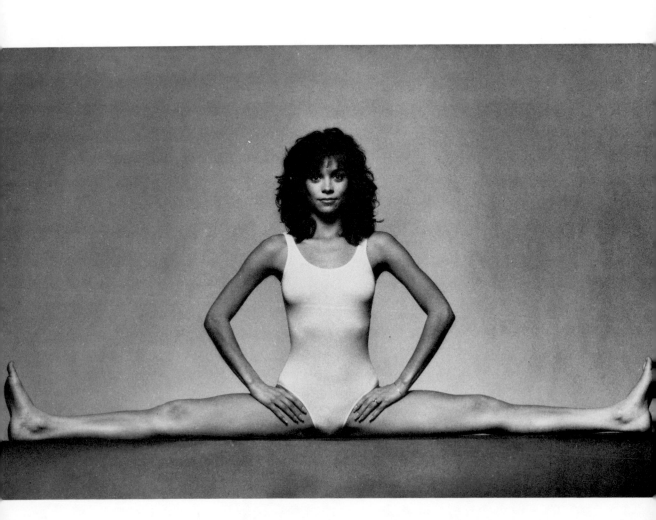

(2) Place hands on the floor in front of you. Take a full breath in and on exhalation, walk hands out in front of you, stretching forward from the hips.

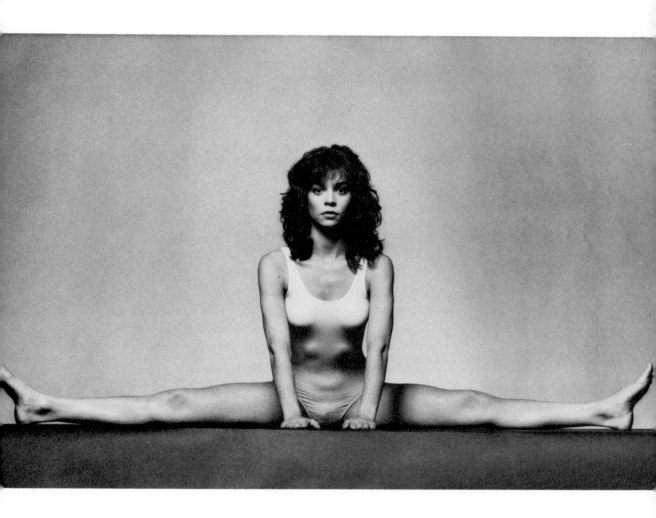

(3) Work at placing abdomen on the floor, then chest, and then chin. Breathe through for 10 breaths.

Moves Out:

Slowly walk hands back, pressing torso back up tall. Bring legs together. Take a full breath in through the nose and out through the mouth.

Be Aware: Go only as far as your flexibility allows. Tighten the front of your thighs and press your seat bone behind you, giving you the correct extension from the hips without bending into your spine. Keep kneecaps facing as much as possible toward ceiling.

Benefits: Stretches the hamstring muscles and side torso muscles. Teaches the mind to surrender its restless, complaining ways; creates a quiet world within.

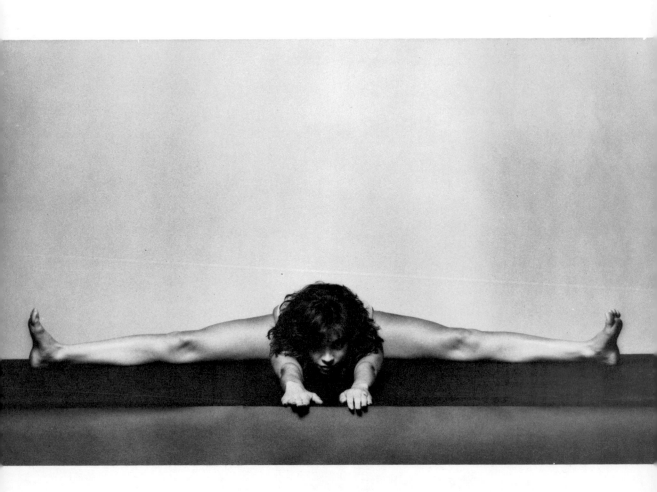

Sitting Angular Pose with Partner

Moves In:
(1) Sit facing partner with legs stretched apart, the soles of your feet touching those of your partner.
(2) Stretch arms out and hold each other's wrists.
(3) As one partner lies back on the floor the other is pulled forward, his stomach between his legs.
(4) Reverse positions.

Moves Out:
Both partners sit up straight and take a full breath in through the nose and out through the mouth.

Be Aware: Be gentle with partner. Bend from the hips, not from lower back.

Benefits: Same as the Sitting Angular Pose, except the stretch is intensified.

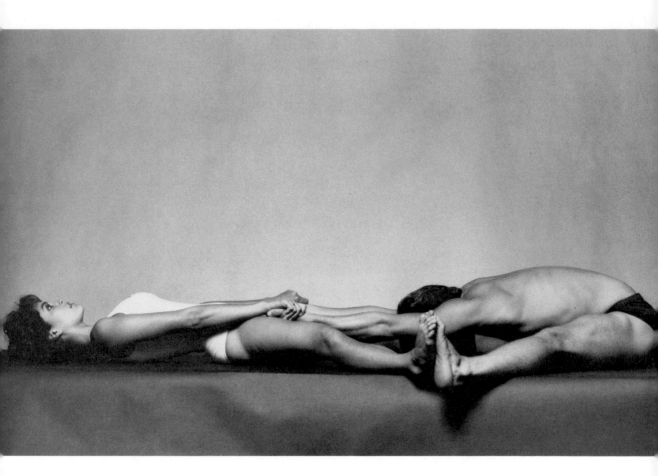

Butterfly Pose

Moves In:

(1) Sitting on the floor, bend your knees, bringing the soles of your feet together. Interlace fingers around toes and pull heels as close to body as possible. Bounce the knees gently to loosen legs.

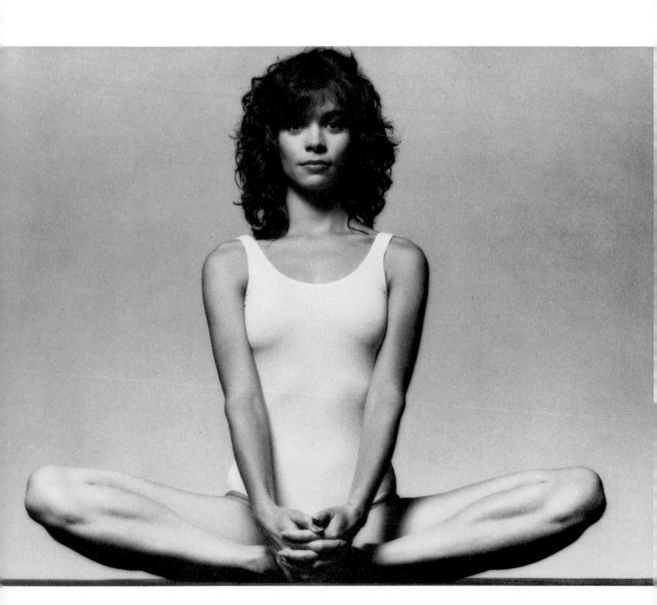

(2) With hands on either knee, press them as close to the floor as possible.

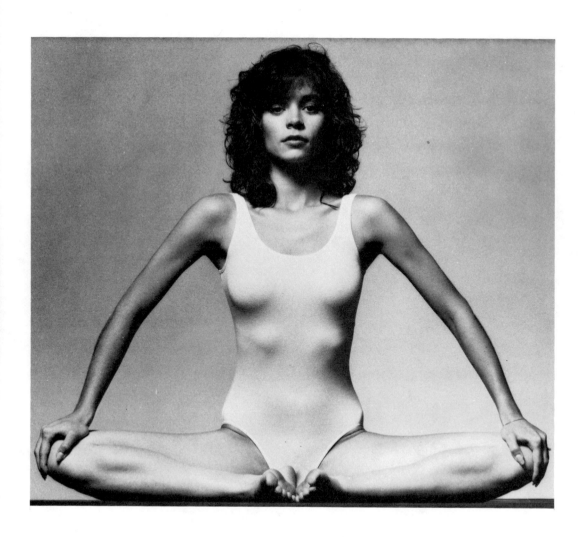

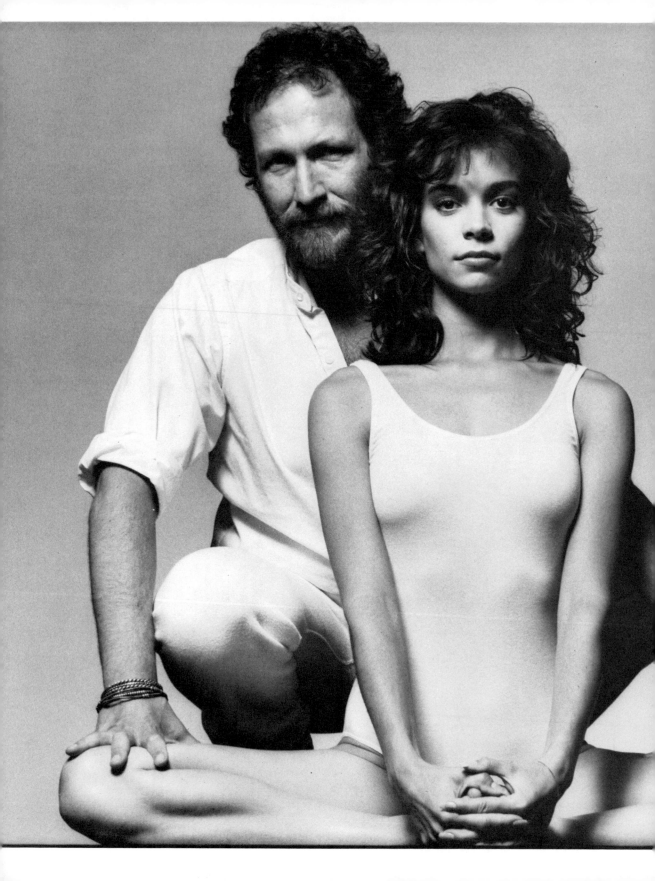

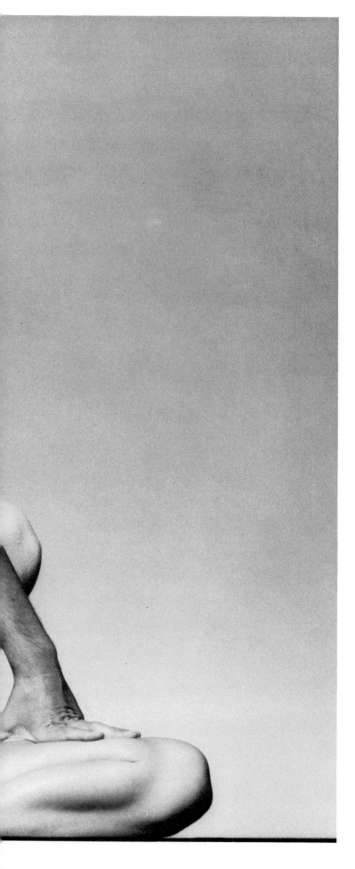

(3) If there's someone around, let him or her assist you.

Moves Out:

Stretch legs straight out in front of you, bouncing them gently to release any pressure.

Be Aware: Keep spine absolutely straight. (If you can't, sit up against a wall and then press knees down.)

Benefits: Releases tension from abductor muscles, healing knee disorders. Removes sexual inhibitions. Keeps hip joints loose and massaged.

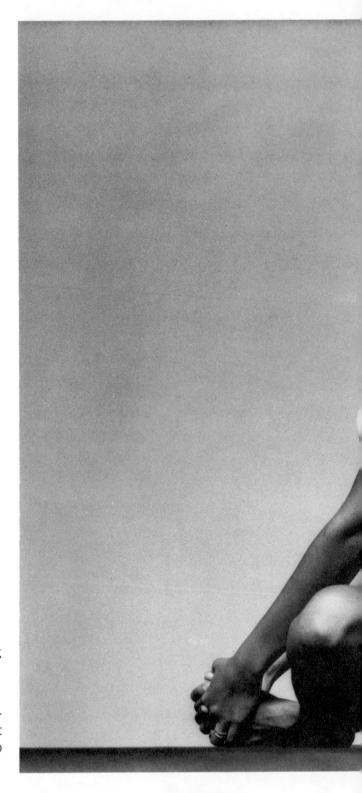

Butterfly with Partner

Moves In:
  (1) Sit back-to-back with part-
      ner, the soles of your feet
      together. Pull heels into
      body.

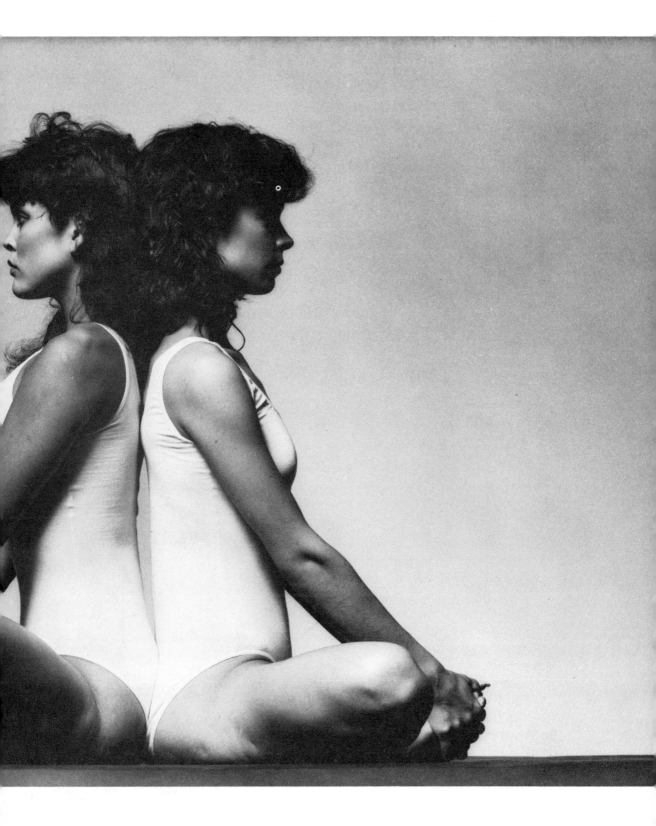

(2) Reach back and place your hands on your partner's thighs. Press his or her legs gently down toward the floor. Then reverse. Remember to breathe through the stretch.

Moves Out:
Stretch legs out straight and gently bounce them on the floor.

Be Aware: Keep spine tall. Be gentle with partner's legs!

Benefits: Working with a partner gives you the leverage necessary to get your knees as close to the floor as possible.

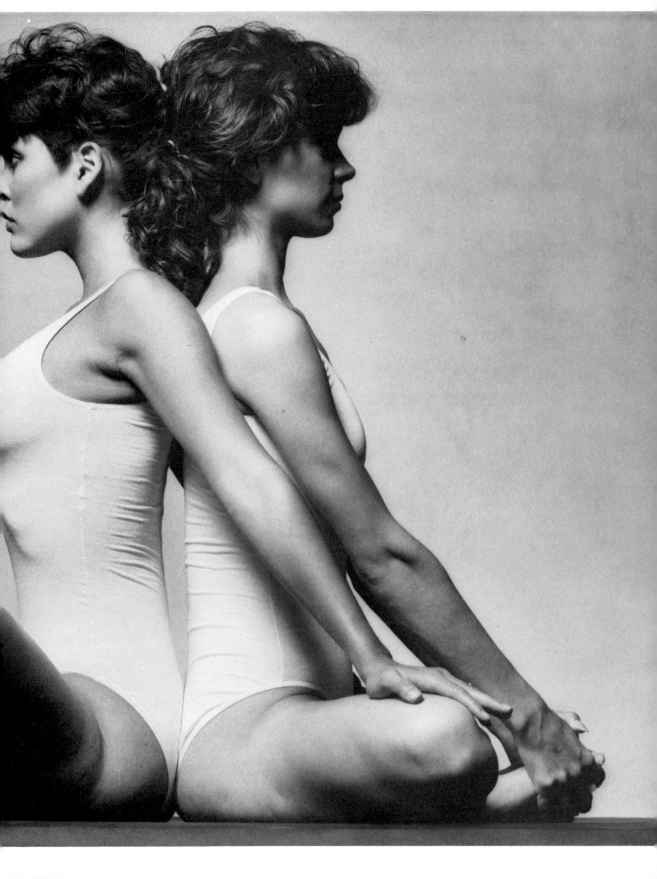

LOTUS SEAT

Human beings sit naturally cross-legged on the floor. It is therapeutic, as it keeps the hips supple and correctly aligned. The hips are the foundation of the spinal column, the central cord of your nervous system. At first, your hips may be stiff, which causes your spine to bend, making the position most uncomfortable. If so, sit on a firm cushion or on a telephone book.

There are three different seats, ranging from elementary (Free Seat) to intermediate (Single Lotus) to advanced (Double Lotus). Don't hurry! Sit as long as it is comfortable the first day and gradually increase the time.

A true yogi should be able to sit completely still for hours. The longer you can sit still on the outside, without moving at all, the stiller the mind becomes.

So get the ants out of your pants and learn to sit still.

Free Seat

Moves In:
    (1) Sitting on the floor, cross your legs.
    (2) Using your hands, position your buttocks equally on the floor, so that your spine is at a right angle to the floor. Sitting on a phone book may be helpful.

Moves Out:
    Stretch your legs out in front of you and bounce your knees out gently on the floor.

Be Aware: If you have a cartilage disorder in your knee or if there is pain in your knee, use a cushion under your thighs to support your legs. Be sure that your spine is straight (sitting on the edge of a book or pillow will assist you in this).

Benefits: Keeps your legs supple and takes away tiredness. As you sit in this seat, blood massages the anus and genital area. It revitalizes the major nerve areas located at the base of the spine.

It is excellent in massaging the lower intestines and bowels, promoting good stomach movement.

Sit in this posture as often as you can.

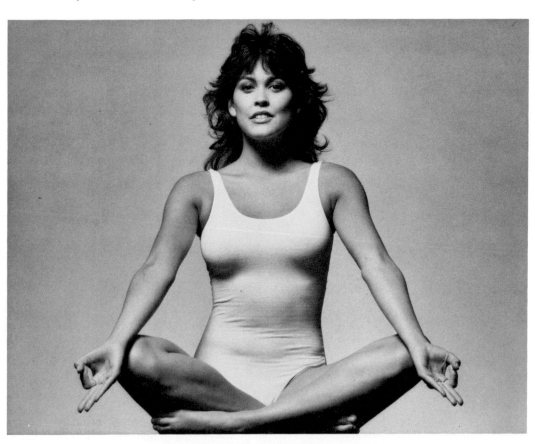

Single Lotus

Moves In:
    (1) Sit cross-legged on the floor.
    (2) Pull one heel into your crotch area.
    (3) Take your other foot and place its heel on top of the other with the toes between the calf and thigh of the other leg.
    (4) Get your seat correctly positioned so that your hips are at a 90-degree angle to the ground. Your spine is tall.

Moves Out:
    Stretch legs out in front of you and bounce them gently.

Be Aware: Don't strain your knees. The hip joint has to loosen to allow the leg to rotate from the hip joint. Keep spine straight.

Benefits: Same as those of the Free Seat.

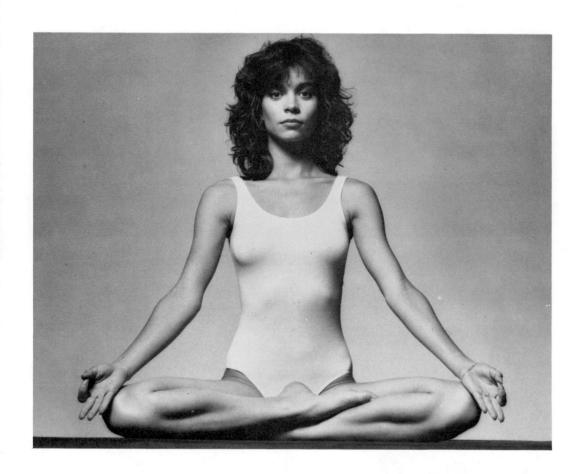

Double Lotus

Moves In:
(1) Sit cross-legged on the floor.
(2) Take one foot and place it into the thigh of the other leg.
(3) Take the other foot, bring it up off the floor and place it into the other thigh so that the legs are folded as in the photo.
(4) Make sure that your hips are positioned at a 90-degree angle to the floor.

Moves Out:
Slowly come out of the position, stretch your legs out and bounce them gently on the floor. Rotate your feet in a circle in both directions.

Be Aware: Do not put stress on your knees. The rotation of the leg comes from your hip.

Benefits: Offers a more intense massage than the other Lotus Seats. It has a profound effect on relaxing your nerves.

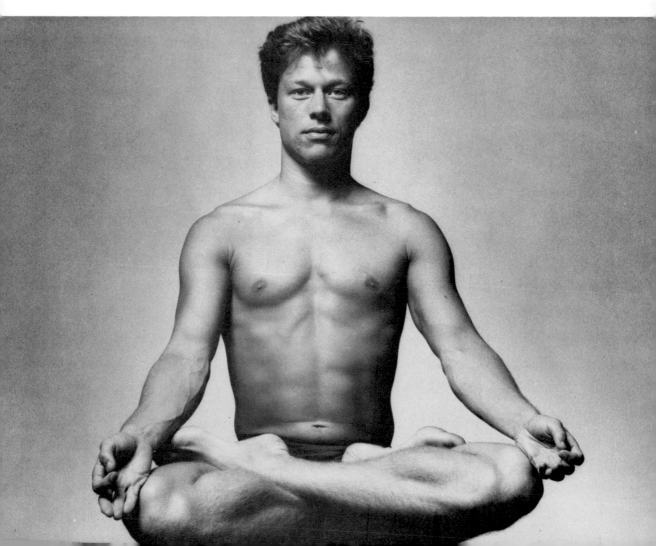

Bellows Breath

This is a breathing exercise which teaches you to breathe deeply and fully.

Moves In:

(1) Sit either cross-legged or in a Lotus Seat, spine erect. Inhale.

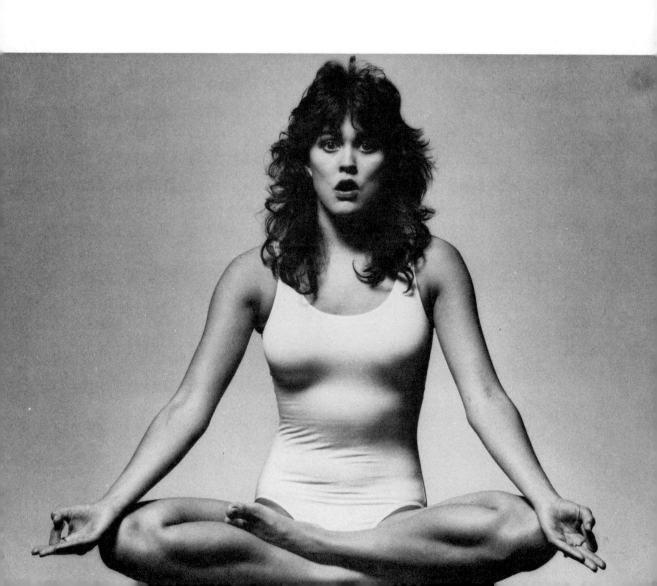

(2) As you breathe out, through your mouth, feel as if you're blowing out a candle flame and your stomach is kicking in.

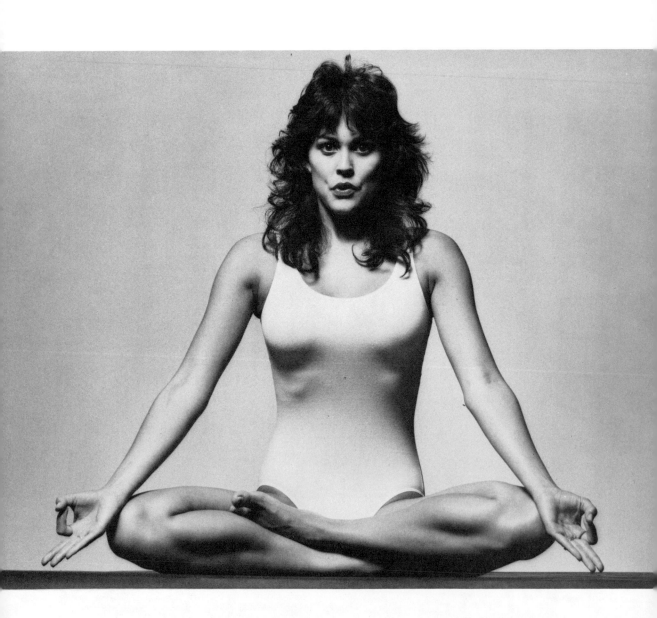

(3) Allow the inhalation to take care of itself through the mouth. (Stomach goes out.) Repeat this breathing in and out like a bellows, starting with 12 breaths and build up eventually to 108 breaths.

Be Aware: For concentration, look at a point in front of you.

On completion, you may experience lightheadedness. Don't be alarmed! Close your eyes and allow your attention to settle in the space between the top of the head and the brain, and you'll feel a tremendous floating, light feeling, releasing tension from your being.

Benefits: Breathing fully and deeply oxygenates and changes the blood.

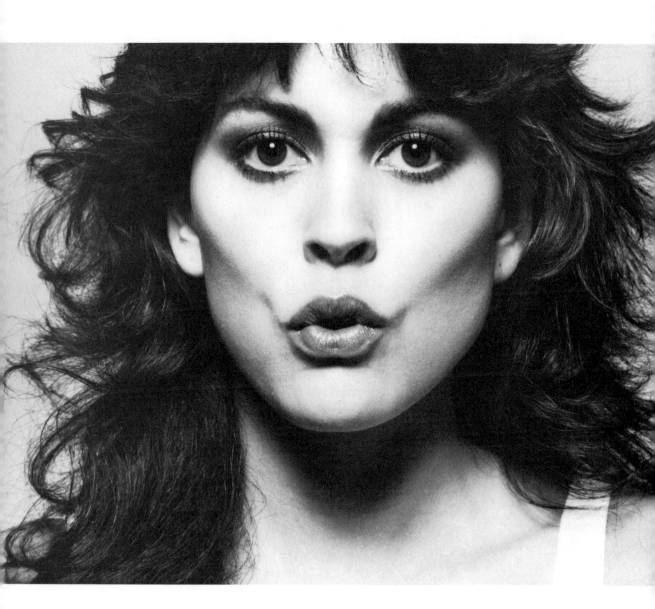

Triple Lock

This is a breathing technique to energize and vitalize your body, mind, and nervous system.

Moves In:

(1) Sit in one of the three Lotus Seats (pages 164–166). Complete the Bellows Breath exercise.

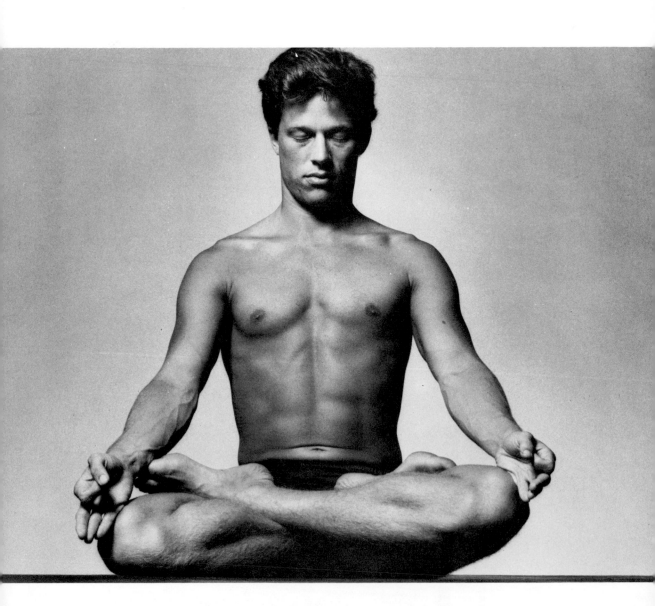

(2) Take in a full breath. First the abdomen fills and then the breath fills up the chest.

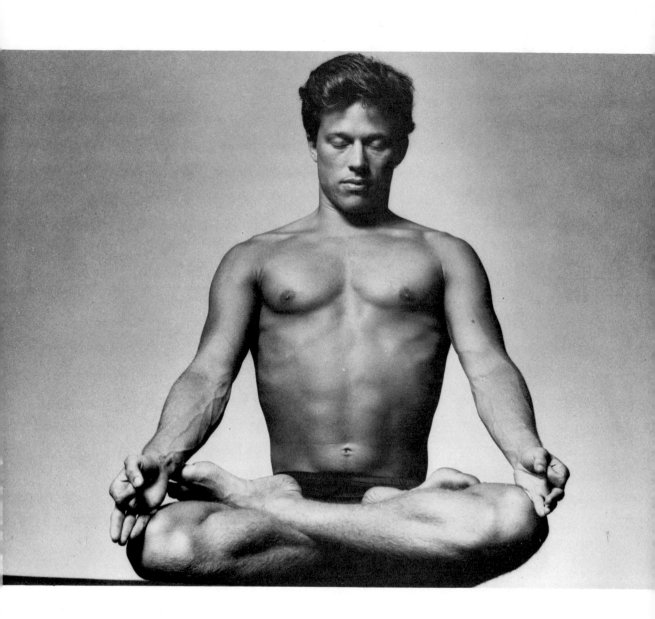

(3) Hold your breath by locking your chin into the neck and chest, pinching your seat tightly together so the anus pulls up, and flattening the abdominal wall. Hold your breath with this triple lock for as long as possible.

Moves Out:

When you can't hold it any longer, break the locks and breathe out slowly, feeling energy rising up your spine into your brain, giving you a light, energized feeling.

Be Aware: When you hold your breath during the triple lock, keep your spine tall. Don't be aggressive. Be graceful!

Benefits: Improves breathing, heals lungs, makes the mind tranquil, gives you an invigorated feeling.

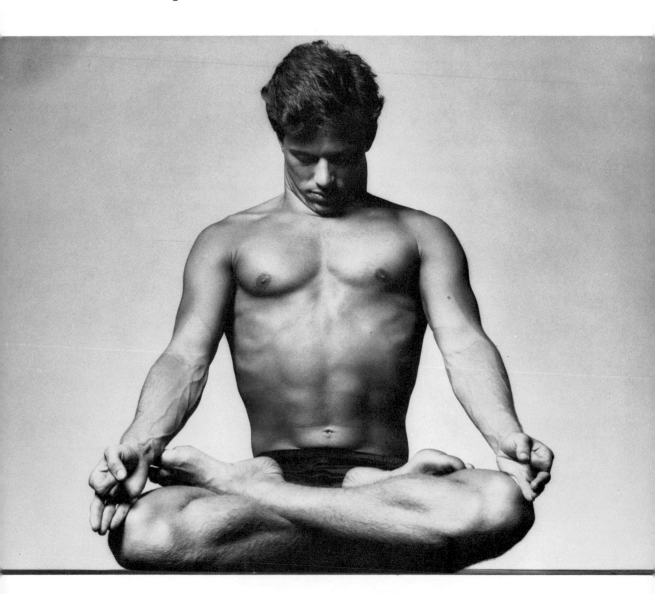

MEDITATION

The Yogis discovered various energy fields that they call *chakras.* In the body these chakras govern and affect your life. Certain colors and sounds activate these fields, charging and changing your energies. Medical science is slowly coming to realize the powerful effect that visualization has on the human being, using both color and sound.

This visualization technique will assist you in directing your inner journey to health, happiness, strength, and peace.

Preparing for Meditation

- It is easiest to meditate when your body is relaxed. So, first do some of the postures or the deep-breathing exercises.
- Find a quiet place where you will not be disturbed.
- Meditate before you eat.
- The more you meditate the less restless you become, so sitting for longer periods of time becomes easier.
- The spine is the central core of your nervous system and must be kept straight. Placing a cushion under your seat bone while meditating will assist you.
- Keeping your eyes closed helps you to concentrate and explore your inner being.
- If your mind wanders, take a full breath in through your nose and out through your mouth, then settle back to meditating.

Visualization Technique

(1) Sit in a cross-legged position or in the Lotus Seat. At first you may need to support your back. Sitting up against a wall will work—or put a cushion under your seat. This puts your hips in the correct position.

(2) There are numerous energy centers (or chakras) in your being. Certain colors activate, charge, and balance these centers, bringing out your positive qualities.

(3) Visualizing these colors in meditation will assist you in a total centering of your being.

(4) To charge your chakras, feel a radiance of white light entering through the top of your head and moving down to the base of your spine, opening the central core of your spine.

(5) At the base of your spine visualize a red light, giving you vitality.

(6) At the top of your sacrum bone visualize orange light, charging you with sexual energy.

(7) At the navel center visualize yellow light, balancing the dual qualities—likes and dislikes, introversion and extroversion—of your mind.

(8) In the region of your heart visualize a green light, balancing your emotions, giving love and compassion.

(9) At the throat center visualize a blue glow of light, eliminating fear and allowing you to communicate.

(10) In the center of your brain visualize a violet glow, bringing you peace and tranquillity, giving the sensation of your brain opening like a soft white flower, radiating light.

(11) Having balanced the energy of your being, focus your attention between your eyebrows, bringing yourself to the center of inspiration and insight.

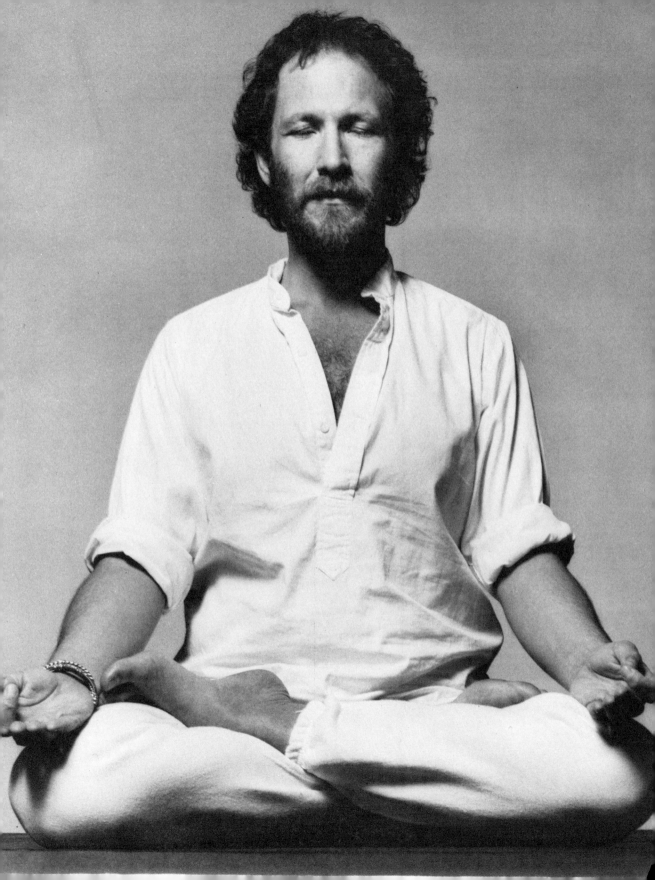

Each of you is a star in your own galaxy,
A sun in your own universe.
Having set your spirit free, feel yourself rise
        to a new and exciting dimension
        filled with joy and ecstasy.
Take this joy into the world with you!

                Hari Om
                Feel the strength within.